Caeia March was born in the Isle of Man in 1946 and grew up in industrial South Yorkshire. She went to London University in 1964 and graduated in social sciences. She has had ME for nine years. As a result of this she left London in 1990 – where she had been a tutor of women's studies and creative writing – and settled in Cornwall. She has published poetry, short stories and non-fiction articles, but is best known for her much-loved novels for women, all published by The Women's Press: *Three Ply Yarn* (1986); *The Hide and Seek Files* (1988); *Fire! Fire!* (1991); *Reflections* (1995); and *Between the Worlds* (1996).

Caeia March has two sons aged 24 and 26. She lives in West Penwith with her partner and two cats.

Knowing ME

Women Speak about Myalgic Encephalomyelitis and Chronic Fatigue Syndrome

Caeia March, editor

First published by The Women's Press Ltd, 1998
A member of the Namara Group
34 Great Sutton Street, London EC1V 0DX

Collection copyright © Caeia March 1998

The copyright in each of the pieces in this collection remains with the
original copyright holder.

The right of Caeia March and the contributors to be identified as the
joint authors of this work has been asserted by them in accordance
with the Copyright, Designs and Patents Act 1988.

The editor has the intention of ensuring that this book will be made
available on audio cassette.

British Library Cataloguing-in-Publication Data
A catalogue record for this book is available from the British Library.

ISBN 0 7043 4539 0

Typeset in Trump Medieval by FSH London
Printed and bound in Great Britain by Cox & Wyman

Contents

Part One: Diagnosis, Definitions and Decisions

Part Two: Family, Friends and Community

Part Three: Healing Ourselves

Part Four: Benefits, Rights and Beyond

Permissions

Aspen's pieces have been previously published as follows: 'Smile Sandwich' and 'Lost' appeared in *Disability Arts Magazine*. 'Lost' also appeared in *Rainbows in the Ice: Poetry by Disabled Writers* (Commonword) and 'Smile Sandwich' appeared in *Dykes, Disability and Stuff*. 'Loving Woman' has appeared in *Hikane, The Capable Woman*. 'Winter' was published by *Disability Arts in London Magazine*. 'Muscle Fetish' appeared in *Sinister Wisdom*, no. 50 and *Pushing the Limits: Disabled Dykes Produce Culture* edited by Shelley Tremain (Women's Educational Press). 'Still Life' by Maria Jastrzębska was published in *Interaction: The Journal of Action for ME*. 'The CFIDS Diet' by Sharon Wachsler appeared in *Ragged Edge Magazine*, March/April 1998.

Acknowledgements

I would like to thank my partner Cheryl Straffon first of all, because we fell in love when I already had ME and we have shared together the ups and downs of ME for the past six years. Thanks Chell for your good humour, love and affection, as we look forward to years of creativity, happiness and fun together.

My deep thanks to my long-standing friends Penny Holland, Pat Hextall and Keri Wood, and my sister Valerie, for all your years of reliability and believing in me, with or without ME. In your very different ways you have supported me through ME, and my life is richer for knowing you.

To my sons Mark and Robert, my thanks for family life and for your unique and sustained willingness to deal with the issues of having a mother with ME. It gladdens my heart.

To Dr Barbara Jacobs of south-east London I offer my respect for your knowledge and your speed of diagnosis. Thank you for listening to me and recognising ME. Without your early diagnosis I might have descended into despair at what was happening. Instead I was able to name myself as a woman with ME and get on with the process of learning about it. I have wanted to thank you for a long time.

Thank you to The Women's Press for undertaking this project and for your combined commitment to publishing books by women with disabilities. Without publishers it is very difficult to have a public voice. Without voices we are confined to the margins yet again.

To Marcia White, London based journalist, I owe a large debt of gratitude for many hours of background research, useful discussions and networking for contributors.

To Veronica Marris for sending me a copy of *Lives Worth Living*. The concept inherent in the title of your anthology on chronic illness encourages me, and it validates us all and makes us real.

Thank you to the ME Association and the pressure group 'Action for ME', for years of campaigning. As you rightly acknowledge, we still don't know what causes ME and we still don't fully understand it. But we will, eventually! Your work gives us strength to live with ME. The fact that you are there makes it easier, because we know that we aren't facing this alone. In particular I thank you for your insistence that ME is not a psychological illness, whilst acknowledging that it can have psychological effects as we try to come to terms with its impact on our previously active lives.

Thank you to all those in the telephone network that I was part of when I lived in London; to friends who have helped me move house and given me lifts and places to rest in the daytime; to Bernadine Evaristo for practical support with my writing; to Lydia Nightingale, Shelley Pielou and Meg Torwl for help with the resources list; and to Marcia White, Lee Green, June Eaton and Jo O'Farrell for useful discussions on women's health.

Finally, thank you to all the contributors in this collection for your enthusiasm for this book. Your flexibility and honesty, and your patience throughout the project helped it through all its stages. Long life and good health to you all!

Introduction

In late twentieth-century Britain, despite a magnificent array of technology bringing us cultural, commercial, medical and scientific rewards, the human body is sometimes still a baffling entity.

In the diagnosis of disease in Britain over the last thirty or forty years, a particular combination of pathological physiological responses has come to be recognised and named. In the fifties it was called Royal Free Disease because many of the staff at the Royal Free Hospital in London all seemed to exhibit similar symptoms. In the eighties, amidst increasing public awareness, it came to be renamed as Myalgic Encephalomyelitis: a collection of symptoms in the human body's immune, neurological and endocrine systems which, taken together and documented over the entire population of Britain, could be called a syndrome. The familiar initials are ME.

The puns on me and ME are obvious, plentiful and nothing new to us in the nineties. When I was first diagnosed, I sat in the GP's office, vaguely familiar with bits of the whole name. So, the diagnosis which saved my sanity, giving me a label for my fearsome set of symptoms, also gave me an interest in the name: ME.

Back home, I found the component parts of the name in *Chambers Technical Dictionary* as follows:

Myalgia meant muscle pain; Encephalomyelitis was a diffuse inflammation of the brain and the spinal cord.

At that time the name ME, with its above meanings, felt 'right' for me. I had experienced the previous four months of ME as if there had been a cold boiling of the spinal fluid so that my brain was turning into a cold pickled mixture of cabbage, cauliflower and anything else that couldn't think clearly, logically or quickly. I feared for my once fantastic memory, which had been fast, accurate, photographic and generally praiseworthy. I also had continuous pain – in every joint and muscle. I felt as if my very DNA was going to unravel with the discomfort of it. The fatigue was like nothing I had ever before experienced in my life.

But the name, however important, arose from the medical knowledge of the nineteen seventies and eighties; and now, in the late nineties, things are changing in the fields of neurology, endocrinolgy and immunology, and it is becoming out of date. For example, it has been suggested that encephalomyelitis may be an inaccurate assessment of the pathology, and as research progresses in all fields related to the syndrome (including muscle pain research), the name ME may have to be changed to something that more accurately reflects the current medical knowledge.

Meanwhile ME is causing suffering, and because one obvious symptom is the debilitating, seemingly endless fatigue, after minimal exertion, it has become linked with other fatigue diseases under a general umbrella term borrowed from the USA. In the USA the collection of symptoms is called Chronic Fatigue and Immune Dysfunction Syndrome: CFIDS. Here the abbreviation that has been adopted is a simplified one, CFS, which stands for Chronic Fatigue Syndrome.

In addition, in those cases where the syndrome develops after the initial onset of a virus, some doctors use the term Post Viral Fatigue Syndrome. However, it is also recognised that not all cases of ME begin with a viral infection. Recent discussion has focused on the relationship between ME and organophosphates, because some of the symptoms of ME are similar to some aspects of Gulf War Syndrome and to symptoms of farmers who have been using sheep dip, e.g. in the Outer Hebrides.

Therefore, ME is only one kind of chronic fatigue. There are several others, and more knowledge is being gained about them at the present time. We have used both names here in this book because one, ME, may be changed over time, whilst the other, CFS, is not specific enough nor currently in wide enough public awareness to be useful by itself.

There are over 100,000 people with ME in this country at present, and very few of them have the energy for campaigns, demonstrations, and publicity events, though some of the contributors to this book have become active within the Disability Rights movement. But here our voices are raised through our writings, as we face the many challenges of ME.

For myself, ME became Middle Earth – an inner landscape of wild moorlands, raging rivers, high cliffs, soft valleys, gentle streams and peaceful woodlands. Its ever changing climate gave rainshadows on dry hillsides; the night air was chilly; and clouds passed across at noon.

It became a landseasky place bringing me its gift of time to rest and heal, despite the terror of the early years of immobility. I began to 'know' ME as a fantastic place of great potential, where time moved differently and I, moving with it, could visualise many centuries, and see and hear beyond now to then, before, what was, and today became tomorrow. It became a place of hope – a land of transformation.

Essentially, its challenge was how to make a worthwhile response to the experience of a physically debilitating syndrome. Could creativity be a route through that awesome, strange and unpredictable land? I became determined that somehow there would be a book about ME – a creative response to an uninvited catalyst for change.

The title of this book, *Knowing ME*, is intended to reflect the different ways in which women respond to this syndrome and the variety of knowledge gained by those of us who live with it.

ME is not the same as depression, though some symptoms of both conditions are still being confused by GPs and the general public; it is not the same as menopause, though some women with ME go undiagnosed at the time of menopause, to which all else is attributed; and above all it is not simply about being tired all the time. So this book is a collection of writings by women who 'know' their own bodies, learning about the deep levels where reason and intuition are blending.

Women have always been said to have intuition, but we have often been called unreasonable for what we say that we know. In many periods of history, women have been ridiculed and scorned for being outspoken about our bodies and our health. To be considered strange or to be disbelieved is not a new phenomenon. These days, if we exhibit memory loss, mood swings and muscle pain, sleeplessness and confusion, blurred speech and words pronounced the wrong way round, how easy it is for us to be once again labelled: but this time as psychiatric cases. If we are also excessively tired and we speak of it, then we are soon said to be work-shy, feckless, unreliable and whingeing. We are above all supposed to be able to bear pain stoically, never be weak, keep on working (at the desk, factory bench or kitchen sink), raise the kids, do three jobs and never make a word of complaint.

As women we know that we need clean food, pure water, adequate housing, freedom from noise pollution or toxic waste or dangerous chemicals, and certain kinds of electrical and magnetic vibrations. Proving this is something quite different – and finding the right conditions for healthy living is sometimes impossible. Health is not a luxury; and a healthy environment is our right. We don't invite disease, nor call it upon us, nor choose to be immobilised by it – but neither are we entirely surprised when some of us succumb to it. Then in a dominant culture of wellness, which devalues anyone who is not healthy, we have to face not only our personal illness but also the loss of many rights in our everyday lives.

We live in a fast-moving technological age in Britain. I have always loved scientific ideas and the possibilities inherent in new technologies. As a woman with ME, I am now given many more hours of the use of my hands by having a word processor instead of an old manual typewriter. I do not want to turn back the clock, quite the opposite: I want a world where women's knowledge and the opportunities of science are blended; a world where it is allowable to dream.

If we don't dream, we can't make our dreams come true. We could not have created this book unless we first dreamed its possibility. Confined to bed for the first two years of ME, I dreamed my way into wonderful places and colourful futures. I dreamed a whole novel until I was well enough to write it and get it published. We can learn to write down our night dreams and use them; we can teach ourselves to record our day dreams and turn them into action. To dream is part of our healing process as women and our creative process as writers. For women in late twentieth-century, high-tech Britain, dreaming is an essential part of being alive, and is no luxury. If we want to change things, be it our own health or the way the world is run, we have to start by dreaming the changes.

This is one of the many things known by the women writers who have contributed to this book. We will let our imaginations travel wherever we please, with no limits, no boundaries. We may be ill, so we will dream of health. We may be unable to recover, but we will dream of useful, creative lives. We may be unable to move, but we will dream of independence. We may be unvoiced, so we will dream of being published. We may not know the causes of ME, but we will not give up the dream of funded research until there is no more ME.

In this collection, which began with a dream, there are facts and fictions, poems, articles, letters, diaries, conversations, interviews, rantings, ravings, grumblings and perfect sweetness. There is romance and celibacy, seriousness and humour. I am delighted to be the editor.

This book is one small contribution to the knowledge of ME. It is, in itself, a celebratory and learning process for all of us involved. Like the onset of ME in our lives, it is a catalyst for change and it is only just the beginning. The aim is to 'Know ME' so thoroughly that there is no more suffering. This book is a symbol of hope.

Caeia March
West Penwith, Cornwall

Part One

Diagnosis, Definitions and Decisions

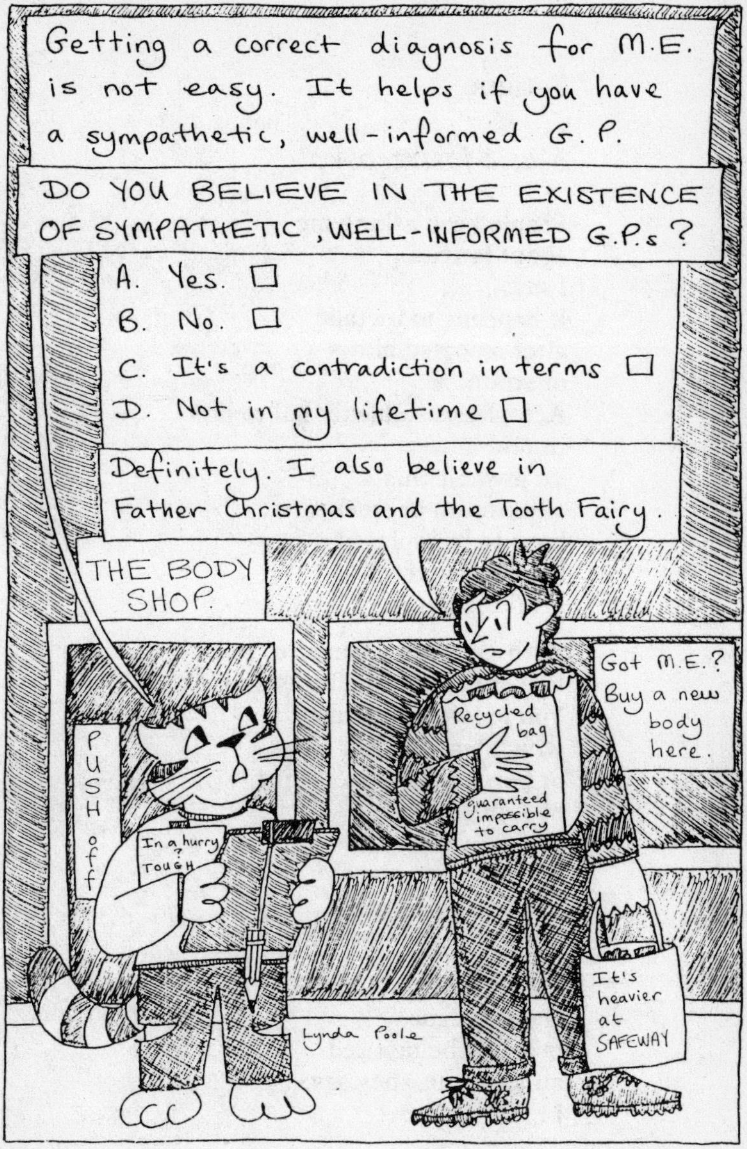
Getting a correct diagnosis for M.E. is not easy. It helps if you have a sympathetic, well-informed G.P.
DO YOU BELIEVE IN THE EXISTENCE OF SYMPATHETIC, WELL-INFORMED G.P.s ?
A. Yes. ☐
B. No. ☐
C. It's a contradiction in terms ☐
D. Not in my lifetime ☐
Definitely. I also believe in Father Christmas and the Tooth Fairy.
THE BODY SHOP.
PUSH off
In a hurry? TOUGH
Recycled bag
guaranteed impossible to carry
Got M.E.? Buy a new body here.
It's heavier at SAFEWAY
Lynda Poole

Fatigue

Maria Jastrzębska

People keep asking me
about fatigue.
I say:
It happens to metals
after repeated blows
or strain.
Aeroplanes suddenly fall to bits
in mid-air.
To prevent this
aluminium or steel parts
have to be replaced
before they reach
breaking point.

With people it's harder to tell
how much anyone can stand.
You're left wondering
which was the last straw
or how the delicate spring
of your strength
got so over-wound
it stuck,
stopped for longer
than you could ever imagine.

People keep asking me
about fatigue.
Is it like being tired
all the time, they say.
I tell them no.

Tired is a shore
I long to reach,
the familiar rhythm
of movement and rest,
the heavy warmth
of my body unfolding
into sleep.
Sleep from which I'd wake
refreshed
shaking strands of drowsiness
out of the sheets
splashing the last little flecks
out of my eyes.
Tiredness can be shed
as you step
into a new day's light.
Fatigue is not like this.

A shadow
no one else can see.
A fog seeping
into my muscles
before I've had a chance
to move –
sheer weariness
on waking.

Clouds in my blood
a dull aching everywhere
and the same acid taste
along my tongue.

Something
I can't pin down
or shake off
altering its shape
and size
but always there.

A joker
pulling the rug
from under my feet
draining the blood
from my cheeks
who laughs
as I wrestle
with thin air.

Fatigue robs
in broad daylight
outrageously,
helping itself
to every precious drop
of my energy,
walking off
with my meagre savings
while others stand by
watching helplessly.

Fatigue tails me
day in day out,
only some days
by pitting all my wits
or by a stroke of luck

and sometimes
when you held me close
I've given fatigue the slip,
laughed right in its face
thumbing my nose at it.
Fatigue is not like tiredness at all.

Duvet Woman
(extract from a longer work in progress,
entitled *Writing in the Dark*)

Evelyn McNally

Nothing works; I am invisible;
no one can see me except the ceiling.
I am whiter, lighter than a feather,
a prescription pad.
This bed becomes me;
I am Duvet Woman,
the pillow, case,
bed cohabitee.
This bed is my mother, my lover,
my husband, my wife,
my iron rations for the siege.
ME is the shadow on the wall
that tucks me in at night,
and wakes me in the morning.

Invisible Woman

Kate Cook

I am the invisible woman.
I am the woman who doesn't have a disability, according to
   the DSS.
I am the woman who has a disability, according to my GP.
I am the woman who has a disabled parking space at
   college, and I worry the staff, because they can't see
   what's wrong with me.
I am the woman who is told that climbing the stairs would
   be better for me, when I wait for the lift.
I am the woman who was told that going to a cabaret is
   boring,
dancing is more fun.
I am the woman who struggled not to help shift the disco
   equipment,
and did anyway.

I am the woman you know, who has ME,
I need you to remember – because I forget.
And sometimes it seems, I need a label for my forehead,
to make ME visible.

Sleeping Sickness

Shelley Pielou

I am a sleeping princess
Whom no prince will ever wake,
Pricked and bleeding from a wound
Unnoticed at the time, since visited in memory
Many times, as if recollection
Could undo the damage,
Unravel the tangled skein of my life
And weave a different fabric of existence.

I slumber on, sleep-hunger now insatiable
A dragon devouring the hours when my contemporaries
Weave rich tapestries of existence,
Work on and dine, connect and conceive
Children they bring to term.
And I dream again of the baby I could not hold
She drifts into my dreams as infant, kitten, fledgling
Grieving my waking.

I age but do not garden my life
It lies fallow and weed-strewn
Showing the faint imprint of past attempts
At cultivation, pansies glimpsed through the couch-grass,
Camellias forlorn to bloom unnoticed
And the relentless slumbering minutes
Ticking by.

I have measured my days in sleep
Not in living. Have slumbered on
Past ungrasped solid joys, life slipping through inert hands
That cannot hold fast, but let the thread slip by
Until I wake, refreshed just briefly.
No longer hoping for the fabled waking into health
But glad of that lesser waking, into respite.

Parminder's Story

Parminder Chadha

I became ill in 1988 but I think that I was quite unwell for a period before that. I broke down in the summer and then the autumn of 1988. I remember I had to come home from work one day as I literally could not move – I felt so ill and weak. I collapsed and had to go to bed. I was extremely nauseous and sick. My body, my muscles, went into spasm. I couldn't do anything, I was completely dysfunctional. I was unable to stand up, to walk, eat or chew. I remember I couldn't even lift a fork or answer the telephone, that's what it was like.

In the first two or so years of my illness I was often paralysed and extremely debilitated for weeks or months. But then I would recover, return to work and relapse again. This was the pattern for the first two years. I also developed other symptoms – severe weakness and strain in my joints and muscles, problems with my spleen and liver, and my digestive system virtually broke down. And at various times I also suffered severely from memory loss, a loss of focus and concentration, and the loss of my eyesight and hearing.

I collapsed four or five times over a period of two or three years. It was extremely traumatic. People around me – my friends, family and doctors – thought that I was severely overworked and depressed. At that time my doctor diagnosed me as having post-viral stress. I also had a lot of turmoil in my life. I was overworked and had a young baby and I was doing a lot of things outside work as well. My marriage ended in 1988 too. It's hard to say how much all of these affected me. I know I would've still got ill but I think I would've recovered if my immune system and my digestive system particularly hadn't been so depleted early on.

Although my GP was always very sympathetic, apart from prescribing muscle relaxants and anti-depressants, there was very little that he could do. I had terrible experiences in hospital and I would never go into hospital now if I could help it. Often when I collapsed at home or somewhere else I would be sent off in an ambulance, spend the obligatory nine or ten hours on a trolley, go through numerous tests, be told that there was nothing wrong with me and be discharged. The medical establishment just didn't recognise ME then. They can't break it down, identify symptoms and prescribe treatment, so they just find it very difficult to deal with.

I was diagnosed with ME during 1989 and 1990 – it was quite a long process. I continued to be ill; eventually I got to a point where I wasn't able to work. I'd been off work for several months then. I'd held a senior post with a local authority and I had to go through their various procedures of seeing the medical officer and even attempting re-deployment when I thought that I was getting better. But gradually it emerged that I wasn't going to be well enough to return to that kind of job again. The whole procedure was demoralising and horrendous because the council's redeployment policy was unworkable for conditions like ME. Finally I was medically retired. This was a terrible shock and I think it was what triggered my depression. It took me a long time to accept being medically retired because I was always career orientated and very active – almost hyperactive.

My job was very demanding but very diverse and interesting. I was involved in casework supervision for social services but I also did a lot of difficult policy work and project development and management. I managed workers and volunteers and I also took part in training. On top of that, I ran a youth club voluntarily outside my job and I was a trainer for the Inner London Education Authority (ILEA). Besides work I had a very active social life and entertained a lot. I really did put a lot into my job. I was probably up at about 7 am and got to bed at about midnight. Often I was still working at 10 pm or doing various things. When I had my son I stopped running the youth club but I was still training independently as a consultant.

A lot of my work was to do with challenging institutional

racism; this has always been the central if not the primary aspect of my work, whether paid or unpaid. I feel that inevitably this was a contributory factor to my illness. Race-based jobs always involve tremendous conflict and pressure – they are inherent in the post – and as individuals, and as black individuals, we often internalise this to our own dear cost. On a wider level, I think that the brutality of growing up in, what was for me, an often overtly racist society certainly affected my immunity in many different ways. It will be very pertinent, I think, to observe the growth of immunity and fatigue-based illnesses in the black communities in the future as our inner resistance wears down.

I first learned about ME from my sister. She was extremely supportive and very assertive in terms of getting help for me and finding out information. She met someone in an art gallery one day who told her about ME. There was talk just beginning at this time about this mystery illness. It was virtually unheard of then and very difficult to address in any way by conventional medicine. As the illness progressed, I learnt more about it by reading whatever little was available and from other people with ME. (People often put people with ME in touch with each other just to share information and look at ways of coping with the illness.) Gradually I learned that there were different aspects to it and it affected different people in different ways and that the symptoms were variable. I became aware of the complexity of ME and finally began to recognise it as a syndrome or a condition rather than an illness.

By 1991 I was medically retired. Losing my job caused terrible devastation in my life as I also lost my house because I could not keep up the mortgage payments. So I went from being very well paid, working and active to being homeless, poor and sick. I kept up my relationship with my own doctor but from about 1991 I withdrew from the medical profession. (I've only recently started to see my current doctor, who's very supportive.) I had to start finding my own way of addressing the illness and healing myself. This process started in about 1990. I explored many different natural or alternative health therapies, including homeo-pathy, reflexology, Chinese herbs, acupuncture and Shiatsu. I also saw a counsellor for four years. All of this has helped me tremendously and, equally important, has helped to empower me as these therapies operate from a more client-centred and holistic perspective. However, costs have been a great issue. It's extremely unfair that very few of these therapies are available on the NHS and we have to pay for them privately.

I feel that I managed my illness in a fairly competent way. When it was clear after about the first year or so that there was something seriously wrong, my sister and I set out finding more about it and setting up a support system for me, finding carers, etc. My friends were also quite support-ive but after a while I lost some of my close friends. Because my marriage had ended a lot of mutual friendships also ended at this time. Two or three very close friendships ended; this was very painful for me, as they were people with whom I was very close. These friendships ended partly because it was very difficult for people to accept the change in me from being very active and competent and productive to being quite ill and vulnerable and needing a lot of support over a long period of time.

If people have a condition like cancer or high blood pressure or MS, something which other people have heard of or recognise, there's a kind of empathy. The attitude towards ME reminds me of the attitude towards Aids in the early days when people either blatantly denied it or got frightened of an illness which they couldn't understand. I went through that experience because I was tested for Aids as people didn't know what was wrong with me. I went through the awful experience of people not wanting to be near me, or touch me or be around me, being set apart in hospital, being stared at – I blocked all of that. Society has a problem with chronic illness, and acknowledging debility or extreme fatigue is a challenge for people because they can't really understand it. They can't understand the scale of it or the persistence of it and what it means to you.

ME is such a debilitating illness; when you're in that situation you need not only a lot of emotional support, but often a lot of ongoing practical support as well. I did get support from many close friends and family for a long time but they got exhausted too, and we've acknowledged that. I've recently begun to rebuild both kinds of friendships again.

In 1994 I moved back to Islington from Chingford where I was re-housed in 1991. There I had joined a support group for ME but it was a counselling-based group and wasn't really appropriate. I found that because I had had ME for quite a long time and had investigated different alternative therapies, I was once again giving support to other people, whereas I needed support for myself. In Islington I got in contact with the local ME network and it's given me a lot of support. For the first time I was meeting people who had had the illness longer than me and have learnt to live with it and manage it. It's made a huge difference to my life and I've made some very good friends through the network too.

One aspect of this illness has been the horrendous devastation of my former life. Another aspect, however, is that it has forced me to re-think my life, and that's one of the most positive outcomes of having had ME. It made me available, for example, to be with and bring up my son in a way that I wouldn't have been if I'd carried on working. It forced me to re-evaluate and re-think my priorities in life. I've managed to work on and off for short periods from 1992 onwards and I've developed different ways of working. ME has actually opened up a lot of opportunities for me in areas that I wouldn't have ever taken risks with before. I began to perform, to work as an artist and writer and to work in the media, in film and TV. It's triggered a tremendous creative and personal exploration for me. It's been the impetus for great growth and change.

What I would really like to stress about ME is that you can't begin to heal if you fight the illness. A lot of people go through a process of denial with ME because it's such a difficult illness and tends to affect a lot of people who are active and are high achievers in life. What has gradually emerged now for me is the fact that I have become permanently disabled. This has become much clearer over the past two and a half years. It has exacerbated injuries to my left leg and arms and shoulders from two road accidents – one which happened when I was eleven, the other three or four years ago. My legs and lower back have become severely weakened as a result of being so ill for so long. I'm now registered disabled and although it's a struggle, I'm beginning to perceive being disabled in a more positive way.

All things considered, I think I've done pretty well. I've experienced maybe four major life crises occurring simultaneously. I remember talking to friends and one of them commenting that even one of those experiences, for example being divorced, is enough to make you severely ill. But for me, I was going through three or four crises of that scale at the same time. I went through so much emotionally. In a sense, I know it sounds ironic, but if I hadn't been so ill I don't know whether I would've survived those situations as well as I did. ME is ultimately a lesson in wisdom. It will teach you many things about yourself and test you to the point of endurance. The secret is to recognise that. I've now learned to work with the illness, to see it as a teacher, and the process is continuing.

Women with ME

Aspen

Without speed, stamina
or strength, with our
wavering concentration
and trembling nerves
with our pain
and disappointment
ambitions vanishing
like tunes in a bubble
we learn
what we can
despite disbelief
claim our anger
lust for life
generous, tenacious
avoiding wreckage
determined as barnacles
clinging to our stature
on storm-cracked rocks
welcoming the moments
of enhanced feeling
infused with serenity
allowing the connection
intense, expanding
spirit full to bursting
until clouds shatter
into brilliant rainbows
revealing
an alternative view

never mind the muscle tone
find the courage

Ajay's Story

Ajay

I was diagnosed as having ME in November 1991 by a neurologist at St Bartholomew's Hospital in London. I had been deteriorating during the previous nine months or so to the point where I was only able to stand up long enough to clean my teeth. I would then be completely exhausted.

During the months prior to this my energy levels were becoming lower and lower. I was a student at the time and there came a point when I could just about get to college and then I would have to turn around and come home again because I didn't have the energy to attend my classes or even speak to anyone. This went on for a few months.

I was not completely aware that there was anything really wrong with me. I was a student in the second year of a degree – I expected to be tired. I was not able to think clearly about what was happening to me. I went to see one of the doctors at the GP practice where I was registered, a couple of times, and she offered me anti-depressants and a psychiatrist – I declined both offers. I was unable to be clear to her about exactly how I was feeling and what was happening to me. But in hindsight, I was a classic case of ME and I think she should not have been so hasty in assuming the problem was psychiatric.

I continued to deteriorate and have increasingly low energy levels. By July and August it was obvious I was ill and by October I was in bed and couldn't get out of it. My friends were now involved and were basically looking after me. By about mid-November they called my GP practice as I was clearly not improving and they could not continue to give the sort of time and energy they were putting into me endlessly.

Another doctor from my GP's practice came to the house

and showed alarm at my situation. She quickly arranged for me to have an immediate appointment at Bart's Hospital with a neurologist and a doctor who was doing research into ME. I went to my appointment via taxi, wheelchair and two friends. When I got there the neurologist took one look at me and asked, 'Have you heard of ME?'

I had heard of ME but I didn't know anything about it or anyone who had it. He considered me to be an urgent case and tried to admit me into hospital immediately. But as I was not a neurological patient – by his own diagnosis – he could not admit me on to his ward.

I was relieved at having had a diagnosis and the sureness that I was not imagining what was happening to me.

The neurologist had an arrangement with my second doctor to tell her the results of his examination that night. My doctor telephoned me the next day and from then on was very supportive and dealt with everything in a warm and friendly manner, providing me with sick notes and other help as I needed it. I was glad that she took my illness seriously but as I was so obviously sick it did concern me that my illness was only accepted when it was confirmed by the neurologist.

As I was still unable to look after myself properly, something still needed to be done. I couldn't walk at all. I could get to my bathroom with the help of furniture and the banister but it took forever and it was only ten yards away. Soon after the other doctor from Bart's Hospital who was doing research into ME came to see me at my house and did a fairly in-depth interview with me.

During this interview I realised he was a psychiatrist. He was interested in my condition and put me on the top of his waiting list for his ward. His general philosophy seemed rather bizarre and impossible to me. I was not in the least bit interested in being admitted to a psychiatric ward for anything! However, the situation was that I needed to be looked after. It was made very clear to me by both the neurologist and my doctor that there were no other possibilities. I eventually agreed to go to Bart's on the condition that they would not give me drugs or counselling.

I was admitted within a fortnight and was there for nine weeks. I did not take any anti-depressants offered to me and I did not talk to anyone about my life. I had my own room and obviously meals – my friends brought me food as well – and there I stayed relatively stress-free, recuperating. I didn't have to think about anything or be a burden to anyone.

I began to get better. I needed two sticks to walk with as this seemed to relieve the strain on my quadriceps (thigh muscles) which exhausted me the most. I was finally fit enough to go home and be able to feed myself – with some help from friends with shopping. When I first left hospital I applied for Disability Living Allowance. A social security doctor came to see me. The only physical examination he did was to listen to my heart through my clothes. His examination only lasted about five minutes. He later reported that I was fit and not eligible for the allowance. The ironic thing was that I was too sick to appeal against the decision.

During the period of time before Bart's and also for part of my stay there, it became clear that I was allergic and had bad reactions to certain foods like wheat, sugar, salt and E numbers. After eating any of these things my energy would be completely depleted. I lived on rice, potatoes and other vegetables, porridge and oats, mostly cooked in water. This actually led to me losing weight and as I was only seven stone in the first place, I knew I needed to boost my meat intake so I included chicken and fish. I also took 3,000 mg of evening primrose oil a day for most of that time. The strong reaction to most of these foods lasted a few months. Now I only remain slightly sensitive to wheat products.

Of all the theories I later heard about ME – it being a virus, it being imaginary, or psychiatric, and others – I have found that the theories advanced by Dr Paul R Cheney MD PhD [Spring 1994, *Journal of the Chronic Fatigue and Immune Dysfunction Syndrome Association of America*] sit most comfortably with me.

He says that a viral trigger or a previous toxic exposure, or a persistent toxic exposure or viral infection, could be the possible cause. There could be other causes but ultimately they all end up evoking an excessive immune activation state. There are different kinds of excessive immune activation and an example of one is an allergy and another is mono-like fatigue.* In its chronic form, CFIDS begins with a mono-like or 'flu'-like illness that rapidly evolves into severe and debilitating fatigue with dramatic loss of functional capacity. Over time there are also severe neuro-cognitive problems. This takes account of all my symptoms, including not being able to think properly. Although I didn't have a flu-like illness that I can identify as the beginning of my illness, I did have chickenpox in 1988 when I was 35, which I feel may have been a factor.

When I came out of hospital I did what everyone said I should do – take it easy, rest and listen to my body. And I think I succeeded in that. For the first few months I was able to be out of bed for two to three hours a day. This gradually increased over a long time. By the end of 1995 I was still going to bed at 4 pm about three or four times a week but I felt I was getting better.

As for now, I completed my degree that I started in 1989 at the rate of about two hours a week from 1994 until 1996. My health continues to improve and I get a bit better every day. I always improved over the years and did not follow the pattern of relapses that is common. I think that is due to the fact that I did not overdo it. I let my body rest as long as it needed to and I continue to improve. I must still remain relatively stress-free and low key. The whole experience changed my life completely. I've realised what is important in life and have hopefully cut out the crap. I am now a full-time post-graduate student enjoying my life immensely – calmly and quietly, but enjoying it.

*Editor's note: In the USA glandular fever is known as 'mono', short for mononucleosis.

Today

Kate Cook

Today is all any of us really have.
But few of us actually know what that means.
I know I didn't.

Today, because I'm having a good day, I can write about the stultifying tedium of the bad days.

When I try to find the essence of what it is I've lost, that's as close as I can get. What I want back, is the illusion that tomorrow is secure.

Karon's Story

Karon Hawes

Until I got ME in March 1994, I had no idea about the condition and the devastating effect it can have on your life. I had heard of the media's 'Yuppie Flu', but this bore no resemblance to my illness.

Until being struck, I had a very busy life, working full-time as a social worker with adults who have learning difficulties, voluntary work and part-time study. Life was going well, I had recently purchased a house and finally felt settled, living with my partner and our pets.

Then suddenly, without warning, my health collapsed. I don't know if it was the course of Hepatitis B vaccinations I had recently completed, which were required for work, or the Nuvan Top spray, which had been sprayed around the furniture to stop a possible outbreak of fleas, or working through with several throat infections and stress. It was probably the combination of all three.

I was on the way to work when I felt I could walk no further, I felt so exhausted and breathless. I managed to stagger into work, nearly on my hands and knees, and was immediately rushed to the doctor. He diagnosed a viral illness and I was given a sick note for two weeks. I never realised that it would be my last day at work or would bring about such change.

As the two weeks went on, I got much sicker and soon getting out of bed was such an effort, that it wore me out. I began to experience so many varying symptoms, such as night sweats, a low-grade temperature, palpitations, nausea, muscle and chest pain, plus much more. The doctor had to be called out on many occasions, as the weeks proceeded. I was given various medications, which often brought with them their own side effects. I was getting no better, and had lost a lot of weight. Finally my doctor had me rushed into hospital, where I stayed for the next month and a half!

I was attached to a heart monitor for the first few weeks, due to a rapid pulse and chest pain. I had approximately 33 blood tests, a lymph node biopsy and various other tests and scans. The hospital environment also caused me stress, as I was on a ward with people who had major heart problems, several of whom died whilst I was there. The results seemed to take ages to return and I had a real fear of my unknown condition. Also I found the hospital to be homophobic in their attitude towards my lesbian partner; my parents could question the staff about my condition and were entitled to visit any time, but these privileges were not extended to her, which caused us both problems.

Once the consultant had ruled out any major life-threatening illnesses, I was discharged, under the care of an immunologist, who finally gave the diagnosis of ME. Diagnosis was a major breakthrough for me, as it at last gave me some feeling of power, to research the illness and join support groups. Then it was (and still is) an ongoing battle to manage the symptoms and learn to cope with the limitations imposed. I still find the relapses difficult and frustrating, and in many ways have learnt the hard way to give in to my body. It hasn't been easy and has brought about a lot of change in my life, including the break-up of my relationship.

For me, there have been some positive consequences to living with this illness. It has made me take time to reflect on the important things in life and value the things I can do. I have made a lot of good friends through correspondence and my local support group, people who I would have never met otherwise. It has also given me the time and opportunity to study with the Open University for a degree in social science, and it challenges me daily.

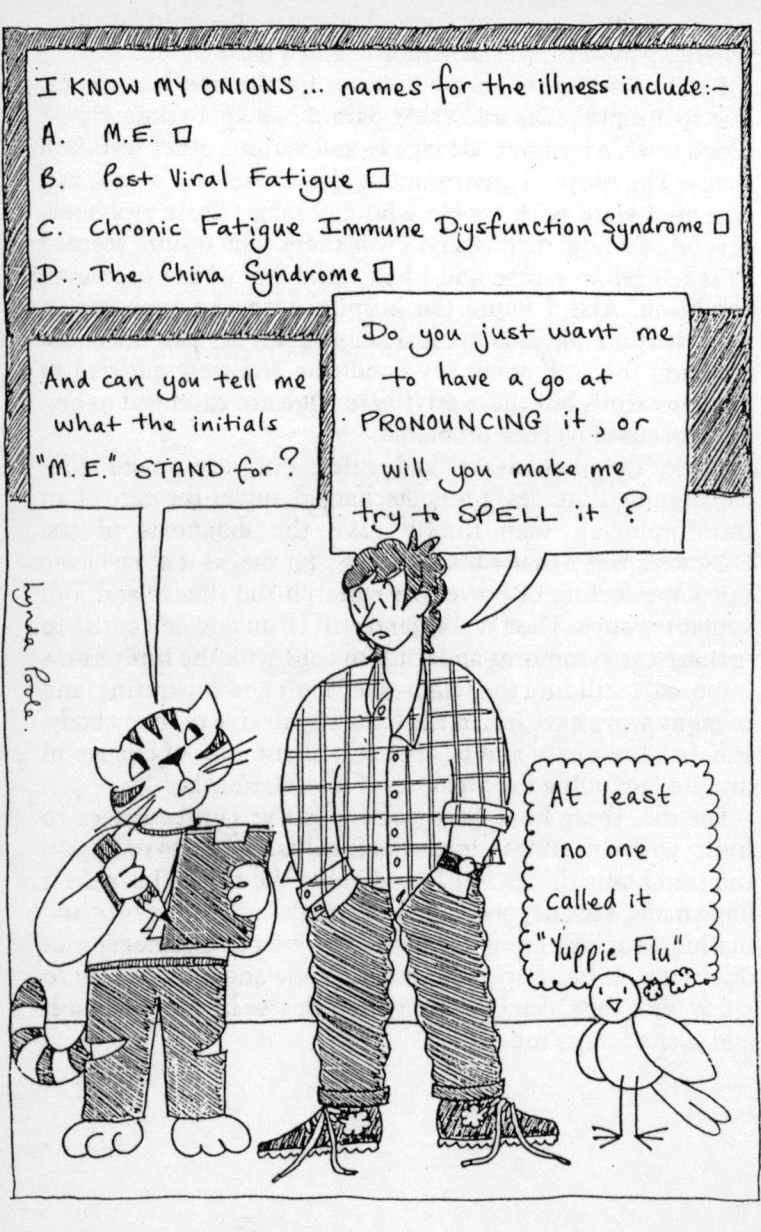

Explaining ME, on a day when you've forgotten what it is

Kate Cook

That's right. It means I'm tired all the time.
No, I really don't look different, do I?
Yes. It's 'yuppie flu' (*for want of a better insult*).

Actually, there's more to it than that, much more.
ME affects me in so many different ways.

I have a leaflet somewhere, you can read it,
and then perhaps you'll understand, a little more.

When I find it, I'll lend it to you, but I'll need it back,
because I can't remember where it came from, and I
might need it.
It'll be here somewhere: I'll find it in a minute. Maybe.

No. I'll send it to you then.
What was your name again?

ME: Is It Me?

Linda Flynn

'What is ME exactly? Is it like tiredness? Is it a form of depression?' These are the sorts of questions I am so accustomed to hearing. Are they really questions of interest; or are they simply an attempt to brush off this illness as merely a cluster of symptoms everyone experiences in the middle of a long, hard, cold winter?

At the beginning, I fought back. I wanted desperately to inform the world that I was suffering more pain than I ever believed it possible to feel. But why? People don't want to hear how a condition can arrive without warning and shatter any hope for the present and the immediate future.

The past is one of the things ME leaves intact. Memories that will never fade. It cannot destroy these moments of nostalgia for me. I proudly reflect upon the days of minimum sleep and maximum energy, of living life to the full without a thought or care beyond tomorrow. Getting up each day was like the rising of the sun; something which was taken for granted. This is a different lifetime, and a different person. This is no longer me.

Will I ever have this life again? Maybe not. Do I want it back? Probably not. ME has re-shaped my life. At first, it completely took it away. Energy, gone. Pleasure, gone. Hobbies, gone. Dreams and future plans, gone. Laughter, gone.

Every emotion – I felt them all. Fear was the first, and possibly the worst. It gripped me, taking over my mind, refusing to let me go. Then came the tears and self-pity, as if I were grieving for a dead friend.

Next, the anger set in like a deep-rooted weed, growing each day, feeding upon the injustice of it all. My bedroom walls towered over me, surrounding me like a prison, preventing me from escaping the clutches of this unrelenting disease.

Lastly, bitterness – a dislike of strong, healthy people who did not have to count the number of hours of sleep each night. Sleep to me was a great comfort; it washed over me like a pain-killing drug, removing me to a peaceful place with no pain. When my brain seized up and refused to function and I could no longer recall the most basic words of a favourite song, or the name of a friend, I felt stupid and stripped of all dignity. In times like this I often wished I would not wake from my sleep; as to me, life was all about high achievement. Grades, certificates, exams. This was all that was important.

But what use are academic achievements to a person who sits like an empty shell, unable to function? Such competition to be the highest student no longer holds my interest. Personal development is all that matters now.

And friends – they were so close to me, but unable to feel this disease eating away at my life: eating away at my soul, eating away at me. My best friends are still with me. I am not alone in my suffering. They too have experienced the brutality of life in their own way. We have all grown together.

My best friend, however, is me. Such an illness isolates you. It transports you to a place you have never seen before, and to survive you must rely upon yourself, as you are the only person that is truly there.

ME has taught me independence, and has provided me with a friend I did not have before – myself. I respect my body in a way I never have before. I listen to its commands and its demands. When my body cries out for rest, I take a rest. I am no longer fighting against the illness; instead I work with it. I must not pretend it is not there; it will not go away if I ignore it, and it is not in my mind.

This is not giving up, or indeed giving in. It is adjusting to a new, more positive way of life, one which is not without its benefits.

ME

Evelyn McNally

I am tired of the word; it is unspeakable.
Nobody knows what it really means.
It is the sickest pun in the English language.
It indicates an unhealthy obsession

With oneself; Freud made a living out of it
Somewhere between the Ego and the Id.
Journalists love it:
ME SECRET LOVE NEST HORROR.

It has a certain ring,
Marriage may not be ruled out;
We have become so intimate,
Holding me closer than a lover's skin.

Enough

Kay Bastin

Sometimes it's
enough
in a day
just to
wake
up

Sometimes it's
enough
in a
day
just to
sit

No clean
knickers
Cat's been
sick
on the
stairs
Pots piled
high
in the
sink
No
can
do

sit
lie
eat
sleep
wait

My Journey with ME

Kate Cargreaves

I am one of the people who crawled out of the woodwork when ME hit the media about ten years ago. Coming across an article in the *Observer* by Sue Finlay (whose initiative led to the formation of Action For ME) I had a flash of recognition akin to a religious conversion. This woman was describing *my* experience, *my* illness, and it had a *name*! This is my story.

I grew up in Sheffield in a happy extended family, within a close community. Life was full of promise. In my teens I went to pop concerts, football matches and dances, and walked in the hills close to our home.

Then I went to Nottingham University to read psychology, and my health took a downward spiral. As a result of persistent fatigue and heavy periods I was treated with hormones for what is now known as PMS. The first tablets had a disastrous effect, and a non-hormonal alternative turned out to be severely habit-forming: stopping them caused nightmares and loss of concentration. The doctor was responsible for not warning me of this, and for his casual use of powerful hormones which was later described by a colleague as being like 'using a sledge-hammer to crack a nut'.

In youthful ignorance of the disastrous turn my health was taking, and of the possible risk to my immune system of swallowing whatever I was given, I felt only confusion and guilt at my lack of stamina. But I continued to lead the chaotic student life – it was 1968 and I was in love!

At the end of my second year, having survived a broken heart, I picked myself up and went off to the south coast to work with a project among the foreign language students. I felt independent, positive, and full of enthusiasm. Within a couple of days I became ill with a mystery virus. I was feverish, confused and tearful and just getting home by train was totally debilitating. I collapsed in my parents' house, where the family doctor told me to rest thoroughly as the virus had 'knocked the stuffing' out of me.

Being young and impetuous I took off to stay with an old schoolfriend, a botany student in Bristol. Each day she dragged me out for long walks in search of plant specimens. I was completely dazed and inexplicably weepy. At night I fell into bed as though drunk, slept around the clock and woke feeling no better. I started the new academic year two weeks late and remained so weak that climbing the two flights of stairs to my flat caused my heart to pound alarmingly.

The Christmas break brought some improvement but I was never again to feel really well. I lurched from one virus to another, and in the process developed a sense of chronic guilt and isolation. Hurtful comments left a deep impression, especially the implication that I was work-shy. Living in flats with other young women reinforced the negative feelings, because it was everyone for herself and a battle for survival. With the benefit of hindsight I can see that people weren't always judging me as harshly as I judged myself, and I retain many friendships from my student days.

When I first became ill the confusion caused me to relive the trauma of the break up with my last boyfriend. So began a long process of trying to link my illness to some crisis, aberration or emotional cause in order to explain what was happening to me. It was a search for order and meaning which was natural, but ultimately destructive because I never did find 'the key' despite being scrupulously honest with myself. This openness also made me vulnerable to the attempts of well-meaning but misguided people to exorcise my ghosts according to their own psychological or spiritual construct.

After graduation I began a teacher training certificate, but collapsed after struggling through a long teaching practice. It was heartrending to give up my career plans. I was unemployed for several months, then moved to London where my health continued to deteriorate, culminating in a tonsillectomy. Plans for a job in Switzerland had to be shelved, and just keeping up my undemanding office job was a constant grind. I would literally stagger home each evening wondering if life was meant to be so exhausting. But at least I was earning my own living. Three months after the tonsillectomy I developed asthma, which I have always felt was linked to the operation or the anaesthetic. I was prescribed inhalers, which I have used ever since. Allergies followed and multiplied: 25 years later, they severely restrict my life.

By now I was well aware that some doctors believed my problem was my lifestyle. I'd moved flats several times, so had various GPs, which didn't help as they never got to know me personally. Ironically, the nomadic lifestyle was more the consequence of my ill-health than the cause, as I was unable to hold down a job or be financially secure. One doctor told me to 'run round the block' after a bad dose of flu. I went swimming instead – and collapsed completely. There were occasions when doctors were downright unpleasant. I was undoubtedly branded a neurotic female which was disastrous for my self-esteem.

I continued to be in and out of work. A job with the Probation Service in which I invested a great deal ended when my senior concluded in a report: 'She seems to be striving for a level of functioning for which her emotional resources are not adequate.' These words haunted me as a damning indictment of my psychological health for years. It was only with greater maturity that I could look back and see just how ill I had been, and how much the struggle to survive in work affected my emotional well-being. I now marvel at my persistence.

The Probation Service brought me some joy, though, in the shape of my husband, but soon after we married in 1975 I had glandular fever and had to leave a new job. Years of striving to support myself had taken their toll, and while other women were fighting for the right to earn a living on equal terms with men I welcomed becoming a 'kept woman'! In principle I believed that equal rights meant the right to a career, but for sick or disabled people the issue was not always so clear-cut. Not having a career became yet another stick with which to beat myself.

Money was tight, but we were able to buy a small house and feed ourselves. We decided to have children and I anticipated a whole new era of bread-baking and Earth Motherhood. Unfortunately my husband was infertile, so we embarked on the ghastly process of investigations, treatments and donor insemination, which were all unsuccessful. Infertility was a deep trauma, as I had always longed for children.

My personal life remained harrowing: in 1978 my brother-in-law died in a car crash and I strove to comfort my sister and her children. Finally, I was too burned-out to keep on working. My husband and I applied to adopt and met with setbacks over my medical, but after a long and arduous process we were accepted and eight months later received a baby boy. This brought profound joy, but also huge demands on my limited physical reserves – our son was, and is, an exuberantly active child. His arrival was quickly followed by my father's death from cancer in 1983. Now, both my mother and my sister needed support. The traditional expectations on women within the extended family put enormous pressure on those who are ill. Had I been able to rest more during these years I might have regained better health, but I do not regret my actions, nor could I have done otherwise.

Life with our young son was wonderfully rewarding, but I was well aware that without a very special partner and the goodwill of women friends I simply could not have coped. Even so, we were determined to adopt another child and despite two rejections over my medical and an interminable wait, when our son was six we received a two-year-old girl. We needed a network of practical support. I had no problems mothering my children emotionally, but regularly needed friends to ferry them from A to B. I read in the paper that a judge had returned care for her baby to a disabled woman, commenting that she was capable of meeting the child's psychological needs, and that practical needs could be met by others. This affirmed me in my conviction that I could be a good mother despite my ill-health.

Another virus in 1986 had brought deterioration and long-term pain across the ribcage (Bornholm disease). It had long been the norm for me to have extra rest each day and to spend time each weekend in bed. I could not walk far nor take part in normal activity, and was ill with what felt like chronic flu.

It was around this time that I came across Sue Finlay's *Observer* article. From that point on I was liberated from the deep-seated sense of freakishness which had been my secret companion for 17 years. I wrote to Sue and was able to borrow books about ME by post. But it was impossible to pursue a formal diagnosis because I was afraid of compromising our already problematic adoption application. Effectively, this meant putting public recognition of my ME on ice. This was deeply frustrating as I longed for vindication after so many years of hidden suffering. But nothing could take away the fact that *I knew I had* ME.

In due course I became free to seek medical confirmation, but it was not an easy prospect as our local surgery had recently changed hands. I considered the implications of seeking diagnosis from a virtual stranger: the fat medical file going before me would undoubtedly prejudice a sceptic. There was a choice of male and female doctors, but I had learned to my cost that a woman doctor was not always a blessing. I decided to approach one of the male doctors as he seemed someone to whom I could relate on an equal level. I wasn't prepared to be patronised; years of battling with the illness and the adoption authorities had made a campaigner of me. The clinching factor was purely instinctive. This man came from South Yorkshire, like me, and I felt he would be direct with me.

It was important to establish credibility. The doctors had no concept of how limited my life was, nor of the endless hours spent resting. I wrote out my story in the third person, for dramatic effect, and made an appointment with the doctor. He looked surprised when I produced my document and asked if I could leave it for him to read, but he agreed. With considerable trepidation I faced him the following week. To my indescribable relief he accepted both the reality of ME and my own diagnosis.

Nothing dramatic happened after my ME became official, but it led on to a successful application for an orange car badge and disability benefits. In the space of a year everything changed – after a wait of 23 years! A fit person may have difficulty appreciating how positive it felt to be accepted at last as 'disabled'. Nothing could alter the years of isolation, frustration, and lost working and social life – nor the effect on my family and friends – but I had learned not to regret what could not be changed, and to value the lessons I had learned along the way. I was, for better or worse, a changed person as a result of the years of illness.

Now, my ME is a fact of life. Admittedly nothing can be taken for granted: only last year I had to fight to retain my benefit. But I am no longer alone, battling against the odds. I still hope for better health, but I have stopped yearning to be a member of that seething mass of humanity known as 'normal'. Watching people hurrying past my window I feel in some ways freed to lead a richer life. If I became well tomorrow I would not, I think, want to adopt what I increasingly see as a damagingly hyperactive pace of life. So much has been granted me, so many relationships have developed which have enriched me, so many insights have been acquired through the long, long years of enduring.

Yes, it would be *good* to do the things I loved and still miss: walk the hills, swim, dance, keep cats. My family would benefit enormously if I were more active, so I won't pretend otherwise. But ME has given me a different perspective. I have learned to enjoy long periods of solitude, whilst needing and relishing short bursts of company and stimulus. Alone, I laugh out loud, without embarrassment, at a private joke or a TV comedy. I can delight in my own company and feel at ease with myself. My spiritual life has been immeasurably deepened, and I have time for friends. This could all too easily have been pushed aside had I been fitter and succumbed to the pressure to do as so many women around me do: juggle work and family, participate actively in school and community affairs, struggle endlessly to find time for themselves, and find along the way that friendship becomes a disposable luxury.

There are still times of frustration, loneliness and rejection, but I am becoming stronger and better able to cope. I am a much more assertive person now – I don't tolerate being put down or underestimated. The women who are my friends now accept me as I am, and don't see me as a hypochondriac or a 'needy cause' but as a confident woman who will take on the system.

Relationships by phone and letter have become increasingly significant over the past few years as I have become less mobile. I no longer regard these contacts as 'second best', but as vibrant and life-enhancing in their own right. My writing is a source of ever-increasing joy and fulfilment. Not only does it fit in with being housebound with fluctuating energy levels, but it has become a positive choice for me. I cannot think of any other work I would rather do. My latest achievement is graduating from an Amstrad to a multimedia PC: for someone who considered herself computer-illiterate, this is a source of great pride.

This account began with a bright, happy child and an active young woman with a promising future. Some of my dreams have come to fruition, but there have been many disappointments along the way. I am now a middle-aged woman, chronically ill, with little hope of ever being fully fit - though I don't discount a miracle. I wish I had not had to endure so many years of illness and misunderstanding, and I would love to be well. But my self-image is quite transformed as a result of receiving the long-awaited recognition of my disability. After years of recrimination I no longer see myself as someone who is 'not up to scratch' but as a woman who, under the circumstances, has done pretty damn well. Mostly, life is good and the future seems bright.

Still Life

Maria Jastrzębska

a blue and white ceramic bowl
of fruit
shiny apples, oranges, yellow bananas
but nothing's that simple any more

with each day of this illness
I grow more calculating
eking out a living
from sums that never add up
the see-saw of give and take stuck
too long
on the needing end

if I bring in the bowl
set it on the table
for everyone to take a piece
if there's none left afterwards
I'll have to call someone
for more shopping
I'll have to ask
all over again
for help

Caroline's Story

Caroline Stedman

This is my journey with ME. Don't take it as prescriptive – it may not be like this for you – but for me, looking back (yes, I'm one of *those*), it had a spiritual meaning. By which I mean it was very much part of my personal growth. A painful, frustrating, at times terrifying experience – yet without it I would not know what I now know about life, about me and about how to live *my* life.

I believe that ME was 'sent' to make me *stop*. There, that's said it (and I don't think it matters who or what sent it, I'm just using the expression). I was one of those people who worked myself too hard at everything; who was always striving; full of 'shoulds'; always feeling responsible for others, and putting their needs (or what they might think of me) before my own. I was loyal, upright and conscientious (I'm still those things, only less rigidly so) and could always be counted on by colleagues, friends and family to do just that little bit more. It's no one else's fault – they just responded to the way I presented myself. And I could be just as driven (some might say obsessive!) when by myself, even if dealing in trivia like playing patience – just one more game to see if I can win – or swimming – just two more lengths so I can say I've done more than yesterday.

Not all women with ME will recognise themselves in this description. But for me it's the nub of things. Our culture encourages this behaviour on many levels. After all, I'm female, I'm *supposed* to put everyone else before myself. I'm working class, I'm supposed to think that the only value on my life is what I do, not who I am. I'm from the 'you never had it so good' generation who were taught that if they only strove hard enough they really could have it all, and by the Thatcherite eighties (when I fell ill) that if they didn't want 'it all' there was something seriously wrong with them. I can remember fighting against these notions on a conscious level at least since my teens, but probably even the way I fought them was overdriven and used up energy without achieving results.

Okay, so not everyone who thinks, feels and acts like this gets ME. There had to be some other factors, maybe even some random element that meant I got ME and the next person didn't. Well, there were other factors – I had a lot of illnesses of various kinds from childhood onwards, lots of antibiotics, steroid nasal sprays, lots of dental work (mercury fillings) and maybe some inherited weakness in my immune system. I also had a very stressful job both physically and emotionally, a lot of stress in my relationship, and 'came out' as a lesbian at the late age of 28. My father died of heart disease when I was only 18, my mother has always been disabled, and I remember childhood as a lonely time when I already felt responsible for the well-being of my family. There were many things that stressed me out by the time I fell ill at the age of 31, and there was too that strange, apparently mild, flu-like illness that I just could not seem to get over, and that six months later resulted in that strange diagnosis ('Well, we haven't been able to find anything else wrong with you, dear') of ME.

And yet only when I began to see ME as a 'breakdown' did I begin to see how bit by bit I could contribute to my own healing. This is not to trivialise the physical symptoms or to suggest that it's all in our minds – I too have battled and raged against that implication. I believe that by the time I went down with ME a great deal of physical damage had been done to my body by the effects of stress all my life and not just in the previous few years. The sources of those stresses were many – physical, mental and emotional – and the 'dis-ease' I now felt was in all those arenas too. What I'm able to say now (after nearly two years of feeling well 90% of the time) is that most of that damage appears to have been reversible. By learning new ways to take care of myself, new ways to think, new compassion for me and my needs, I have gradually, oh so slowly, recovered my health.

I didn't do this alone; I got help where I could find it. The ME group was very important – sharing experiences, knowing you weren't going mad. I also went for healing, Shiatsu and therapy, took vitamins, ate healthily and latterly took cold baths. I learned to detect who around me could be genuinely supportive, eased out those who could not, and found new friends who accepted me as they'd only known me with ME. (Some dear old troopers have stuck with me throughout, of course.) I learned ways to communicate what I needed and not to be too proud to accept what was genuinely offered. One phrase I used seemed to get things across well – I told people I was 'fighting this thing passively' and that seemed to satisfy those who agitated for more progress. I became stubborn and, at times, unaccommodating. I learned my boundaries and took responsibility for sticking to them (though at first I needed help from those who knew me best). I stopped work early-on and learned to keep within my limits – how to enjoy, but not get carried away by the occasional good day or burst of energy. I learned a new timescale: each day was to be enough. And yet also during this time I learned new skills and hobbies – computer literacy, yoga, art – and volunteered for a couple of charities too. (That was an essential part of renewing my confidence to find work.) By now, some of you will be doubting if I was ever really ill – but all this is shorthand for five years of slow, sometimes despairing progress. My golden rule became never to do more of anything than felt right to me. I would no longer override the signals I had presumably been getting all my life of when enough was enough. That in a nutshell is what having ME taught me.

I can still be a little obsessive. I can still forget that only by being true to my own needs can I really make honest transactions with others. I can still get 'ME symptoms', like sudden fatigue or a fuzzy brain if I've overdone something. But these days these things are rare and don't last long. I can never unlearn what I've learned, and nowadays those symptoms just come as a gentle reminder to get back on track. I hope I haven't sounded glib. I may just be lucky that the course of my illness, though slow, included few relapses. But it may also be that I began to get a glimmer of understanding quite early on that I was not powerless to alter that course. I just had to accept rare and tiny improvements, and stay stubbornly moving in an upward direction. Maybe some other life experience could have taught me these things too – I have compared notes with others who, for instance, had bad accidents, or were bereaved early of a partner. All I want to do here is to say that my life post-ME is a great deal more fulfilling, rounded and *real* than it was pre-ME because I now do what I want to do. If you have ME and what I've said makes you angry, because it sounds like I think ME is a 'good thing', or that getting better is easy, or that we must be 'to blame' for getting ill in the first place, then I'm sorry because that isn't what I mean. However, if what I have said gives you any degree of hope, then I am very very glad.

ME and the Other Me

Anna Ravetz

Since I've had ME I have felt that there are two people living in my body. There is a person called Anna, who is me. And there is a person called ME. She has her own agenda, which is quite different to mine, and her own sense of humour. In the early years of this dual occupancy the ME person controlled the whole of my life. She always blocked what I wanted to do. Slowly, the symptoms became less severe and I got a little freedom. But the ME person always waits in the wings, ready to make her entrance. If, in her opinion, I get a bit too much of what I want, she takes over. Then I have to set aside my plans and placate her with rest, rest and more rest.

Sharing my body with the ME person forces me to perform a psychic juggling act. On the one hand, I don't accept myself as I am. I believe that there can be improvement – that either I can get stronger, or that I can make a better life for myself even if I don't get any stronger. I have to believe this. I could not bear my life if I didn't.

But all of us who have ME know that improvement, if any, does not exactly come quickly. I study the ME person in me to see how she works. I fit what I want to do around what she needs me to do. Often, I drop everything and just veg out for a day or two. I hate this, but she loves it. But, much as I placate her, change is heartbreakingly slow. So I have to accept myself as I am, my life as it is. If I did not, I would go mad with frustration and boredom.

Every day, I am trying to be patient, trying to bear the hard things about this illness, trying to accept myself as I am. The mindset required for acceptance is completely different to the mindset required for change. Yet every day, I have to juggle both states of mind – working for change so that I can bear my frustration, accepting myself so that I do not go mad with disappointment when change doesn't come. Now I am stronger it is a little easier. The ME person and I have reached something of an accommodation and I have a little room from her. It is easier to accept what I cannot do when I can do some of what I want. When I was very ill, I found it agonisingly hard to accept myself. My physical state, and my life (with the exception of my relationship with my partner), were just too awful.

Yet sometimes, in those hard early years, I would reach a state of acceptance that was far deeper than anything I feel nowadays. At those times I had a greater sense of peace and self-love than ever in my life before. In the second year of my illness, these moments came after my weekly counselling sessions. It was a tremendous effort to get myself there, and it was frequently the only time I left my flat all week. I would be shattered when I got back and would crawl straight into bed, so before I left I would make hot water bottles and wrap them up well so that my bed would be warm for my return. My cat grew to like this routine and would arrange herself on top of the bottles. An hour and a half later, I would return. In my memory, sun is always streaming into my bedroom. It is midday, which is the quietest time of day there, and the room feels very peaceful. The cat is so deeply asleep that she does not even stir when I come in, and she has not changed position since I left. I am very tired, and I do not mind; I am looking forward unequivocally to giving into it. I slide into bed, shut my eyes, and wait for sleep. I am completely content.

For the past three years of her illness, Monica Shutterspeed has used photography to chart her progress through both the depths of depression and her occasional good days. She feels this exercise in "photo-therapy" has helped her enormously, and hopes to inspire fellow sufferers to reap similar benefits. "I feel the photographs shown below (taken at six-monthly intervals, in mid-winter and mid-summer of each successive year) reflect the inner changes and growth I have experienced as a result of having M.E." says Monica.

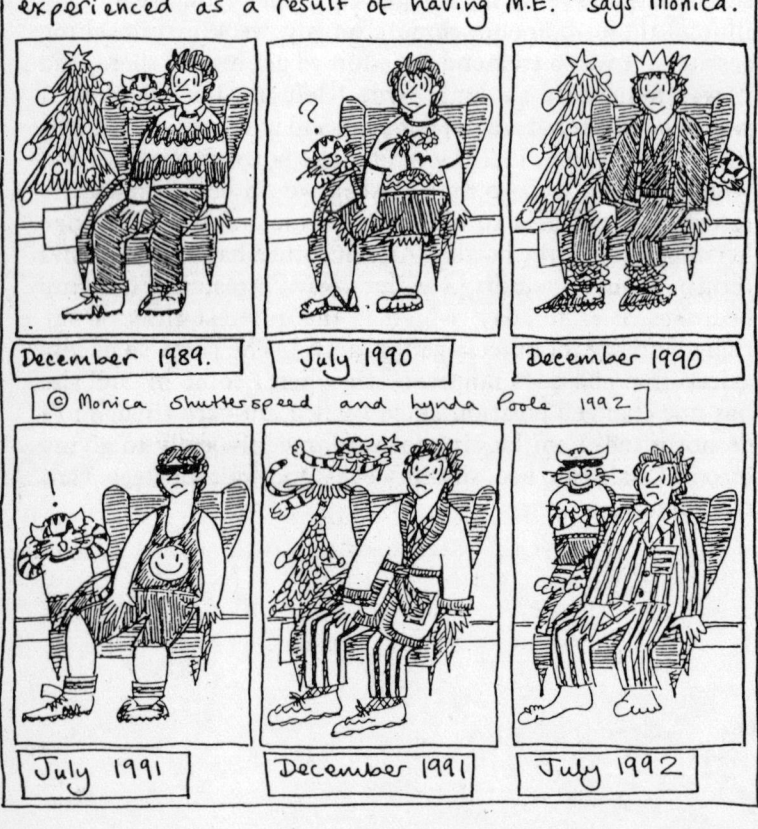

December 1989.   July 1990   December 1990

© Monica Shutterspeed and Lynda Poole 1992

July 1991   December 1991   July 1992

Throw Me a Safety Line

Amanda Cornu

Give me some sort of hope
that there could be some change
A glimmer of energy
An iota of clear-headedness
Just throw me a safety line
And I'll haul myself in
Struggling and pulling
reaching and grasping
For determination and will-power are mine.

Yet so often the rope snaps
I am cast adrift
Left licking my wounds
Shoring up my hope.

Hate is fast growing
The key word
The cornerstone
Of this illness ME
Such a life sucker . . . a leach
Yet it will not . . . cannot
Destroy the essential me
For I am worth
An ocean of pearls
Glistening, reflecting wonder.

What a Difference a Year Makes!

Marcia Francis Spence

I am inspired to share my story for several reasons, not least because I am black and female.

Provision of service for the various groups in society is only possible if we all ensure our needs are identified and acknowledged.

ME is a stress-related illness, and for many black women in my age group (early forties) life has been very stressful. This results in part from the pressure on us to juggle our tasks and make maximum use of our time, refusing to accept the position allotted to us in society; and in part because of the meandering route we have often been forced to take in our attempt to enter the professions. There is, however, a dearth of recorded evidence to indicate the impact of this degree of stress.

Black women appear to be absent in the statistics on chronic illnesses such as ME. If my experience, along with what has been happening to women in general, is any indication then I would have to conclude that the absence has much to do with their being directed towards the psychiatric department where they then merge into the statistics there.

I was brought up to believe that the only way to change your situation was through hard work and determination, and that this combination provided the key to success. I also believe in taking control of my own destiny. Like many women, and perhaps the majority of black women I am not averse to hard work, long hours and working a double day. Until the onset of my illness the luxury of focusing exclusively on one task at any given time had always eluded me. My days were always tightly packed in an attempt to achieve the maximum out of them as I moved towards my goal.

I had been relentlessly driving myself for years, disconnected from who I was or what I really needed as an individual. I had become adept at ignoring many aspects of my life, past and current, that needed to be addressed and healed.

It is not that I was a workaholic but because when you are starting at the back of the bus and harbour aspirations to reach the front you have a longer and more complex journey than if you entered from the front or the side. If you are content with where you have been placed then fair enough, but if you are not you had better be prepared for a ride which is bumpy, with others not only questioning your right to be there but also pushing you out of the way. No sooner have you stepped forward a few paces than you are jostled back, often to where you started. You will have to step out of the way for others to pass by, and you become accustomed to standing still for longer. In the midst of all this you have to be tenacious enough not to give up. Along the way you will occasionally meet one or two individuals with a conscience, who whilst not actually stepping aside for you, will support you in your efforts to move forward. You are however basically on your own moving through a system which was not designed with people like you in mind, and where you are not familiar with the rules. You are attempting to break down barriers; this can be extremely painful and frustrating. This is how I would summarise my attempt to progress educationally and professionally through the British system. My determination has always provided the fuel which has kept me going. One way of making certain I do something is to tell me I cannot do it!

I started my working life as a nurse but soon became disenchanted with the long unsocial hours. Once I entered motherhood a career in nursing proved incompatible with childcare and the costs started to outweigh the rewards. Deciding it would be more manageable to combine childcare with further study, I returned to education, progressing from

'A' levels through to attaining graduate and postgraduate qualifications. Although I had to dedicate many hours to studying, I could arrange my time more efficiently while gathering skills to secure employment when both children were in school. We were all benefiting from this arrangement. I was available for my children at the times they needed me most and I was obtaining the stimulation needed while also making preparation for the future.

However, half-way through my masters studies I became ill. The main symptoms were headaches which were so severe that even my own thoughts were too much to listen to at times. My then GP suggested I cease studying as in his opinion I had taken on too much. I was torn. I felt as if I was gambling with my health but nevertheless I was now too close to achieving my goals for stopping to become a viable option.

Rather than give up totally I negotiated with my department to suspend my studies for a month so I could rest. After this interval I returned and successfully completed the course. This I achieved only by taking things one day at a time and mustering up every ounce of energy I possessed to 'keep my eyes on the prize'.

On completion I embarked on a career as a probation officer. Before long I found this too restricting and, in pursuit of new challenges, stimulation and opportunity for growth, I accepted a post as lecturer in social work at the university of Durham. I made enormous personal sacrifices to go there and fully intended to make it worthwhile. During the four and a half years I spent there I met the challenges and overcame many obstacles while trying to fit in – without selling my soul or allowing myself to be consumed by the ethos of the academic environment. It was perhaps inevitable that I succumbed to the flu virus during my first year. I worked through it for the most part, reluctant to take time out so soon after taking up the post. I was also feeling conspicuous enough without wanting to draw unnecessary attention to myself by publicly cancelling my duties. Looking back, I now identify this as the onset of my illness.

I never fully recovered from some of the symptoms of the flu which remained with me long past its normal time-span. I used part of my leave intermittently to provide recuperation. Leave, however, was an alien concept for academic staff in my centre. I soon realised that rather than using leave for rest and recuperation, which was the norm when I was a practitioner, here it was regarded as the only ongoing space available to write and research. How, I wondered, did others in my field keep abreast of the demands of practice and those of the university?

After two years, during which I had overcome many personal and professional crises, I was feeling as if tiredness had become a part of my very being. I was not averse to working long hours, expanding myself to the maximum capacity in order to achieve my goals. But it reached the point where I could muster up just enough energy to transport me through my working day with nothing left for socialising.

I was always exhilarated by my work but the increasing tiredness was causing me concern. I tried just about every remedy in an attempt to provide relief but to no avail. I was meeting my targets at work but was increasingly encroaching on my already limited personal time to do so. I began to lose perspective, and just at the point where I started to recognise that my life had been reduced to merely work and sleep, I received a telephone call informing me that my father, in Jamaica, had died suddenly of a heart attack.

I had put much of my personal life on hold to accommodate career aspirations but this was one aspect that would not go on hold. Although devastated by the news I could not even allow myself to let go completely and react as I had several stages to move through before I could allow myself the luxury of breaking down completely and acknowledging my grief. For example, I would need to transfer work to colleagues, drive to Sheffield which is where my family were based, and secure a flight to Jamaica. I realised that I had stretched myself to such an extent that there was now no reserve energy to carry me through this major crisis and only sheer willpower enabled me to complete the necessary tasks.

After compassionate leave I returned to work and immediately resumed my duties. After a week I woke one morning to find I could not get out of bed: my body refused to follow the instructions being relayed to it by my brain. I consulted my GP and after much persuasion I agreed to take sick leave. I knew instinctively that I had allowed myself to reach the stage of burn-out and I was very frightened not only of the consequences of burn-out but also of what might happen if I allowed myself to step off the roller coaster which was now my life.

My journey towards diagnosis was then characterised by one battle after another.

I accepted that I was ill and not just tired; the question now was *how* ill? What was wrong with me and how could I make myself well?

I consulted my GP and informed him of my symptoms as honestly and articulately as I could. His response was to diagnose anxiety and prescribe anti-depressant medication. Feeling I had not been heard I responded by disagreeing with his assessment and refusing the prescription. As far as I was concerned the symptoms I was experiencing could not simply be explained as the result of depression or anxiety. My anxiety level did increase, however, as the symptoms persisted and worsened and each test returned negative. The doctor suggested I take sick leave in order to rest as failure to do so would lead to deterioration. It took a few more visits before I reluctantly agreed. I was informed enough to be wary of taking anti-depressants when the cause of my illness had not been ascertained. I knew that it could lead me on to the slippery slope to losing control and being misdiagnosed.

Whatever else happened it was imperative that I retained a degree of control not only over how diagnosis was arrived at but of what treatment I received. Whilst I was anxious to discover what was making me ill, I was adamant that I would not allow myself to be prescribed drugs I did not need and which could produce harmful side effects. My years in higher education, love of books and interest in developments in the black community as well as the impact of those developments, both nationally and internationally, was now paying dividends in that not only was I assertive but I also had enough confidence and knowledge to challenge assumptions.

I was also aware that knowledge equalled power and if I could therefore ensure clarity in respect of what was wrong with me and avoid misdiagnosis then I could determine the most appropriate treatment. I therefore had to be informed and not allow myself to be sedated into passivity. I owed it to myself to search for information in both usual and unusual places. However, this knowledge made it no easier for me to act. Any woman who fits the stereotypes, has a non-specific illness and an assertive nature is more likely to be labelled in a negative way by the medical profession should she dare to challenge them; because they have been encouraged to believe that they are God on earth.

Despite a series of tests proving negative I was having difficulty sleeping and relaxing. I continued to refuse the medication being offered and embarked instead on non-invasive therapies: massages which aided relaxation and sleep; regular gentle exercise followed by a sauna at a leisure club; stress management; and periods of total rest each day. During this time I had difficulty watching television, listening to the radio or music or even indulging in my love of reading as my concentration was severely affected. This was quite a shift from being able to juggle several things at once.

I was on sick leave for four months; and I returned to work feeling much better although not fully recovered. I immediately resumed the pace I was working at prior to sick leave. Six months later I was feeling as exhausted as I had at the point I went off sick. Now I was in no doubt whatsoever that something was very much amiss and it could not be repaired simply by a reduction in my working hours. Despite feeling increasingly unwell I refused to revisit my

GP. I was now exhibiting the classic signs of ME although I was not aware of this at the time.

An appointment for a routine smear test brought me to the hospital. The doctor's response to the reading of my blood pressure, and her fury as she reeled off the risks associated with such a high reading, ordering me to get medication first thing in the morning, plus my realisation of the dangers my more recent symptoms were suggesting, shook me so intensely I sat in my car and wept.

Fear washed over me as I drove home and remained with me throughout the night as I recalled the hazards of high blood pressure from my nursing days. The faces of patients I had nursed with strokes, kidney failure and recovering from heart attacks passed before me.

I was again reluctant to take time off work as advised – a new intake of students was due to start within weeks and we were very short staffed as usual – and chose instead to slow right down. Referral to a cardiologist and another battery of tests threw no light on what was causing me to be so unwell.

A severe disadvantage for me at this time was that my own GP, who had himself only known me a year, was on sabbatical. I was therefore seen by a variety of locums during this crucial time when I was at my most vulnerable. As I tried in vain to convince the doctors that I was ill they treated me as if I was hysterical and needed to be pacified. It became obvious that they were not listening to me or taking me seriously and as a result I refused to follow what seemed to me unjustified instructions, which is how I viewed the anti-depressants they were still anxious to prescribe. It was here that the battle began. My fears about my health were increasing and I felt I had to keep a grip and at all costs retain control over what was happening to me. I also feared for my job and could not bear to tell anyone that I was ill again. I was beginning to feel out of control and that there was no one on my side. At times I thought I was going mad and my fear heightened.

Fortunately at this point I still had a salary and some

savings which enabled me to pay for private consultations in both orthodox and alternative therapy. In my experience, being able to pay for consultations made a significant difference in securing an early diagnosis. It also enabled me to retain my self-esteem, which was fast being eroded by the medical profession. I soon became aware of their often unprofessional behaviour towards me but was powerless to act on it. Some were very hurtful and tried to undermine me, particularly when it came to interpreting the information I was giving them. Being able to pay had the desired effect but I am resentful that I had to pay for treatment which should have been available to me as a right. I am conscious that many women, and certainly many black women, are not in a financial position to be able to take advantage of this option.

I dabbled with various alternative therapies until by chance I came across a book on fatigue written by a naturopath. A consultation with the author resulted in a suggestion that I was suffering from chronic fatigue syndrome. I cannot describe the overwhelming sense of relief that I experienced on having my illness identified and recognised. I now had confirmation that it was not 'all in my mind', that I was not simply tired or lazy, but ill. The relief was curtailed by the realisation that there were no short cuts to getting well; it was going to be an uphill struggle. Prior to this I had no knowledge of the illness and subsequently set about becoming informed. I started by contacting the ME association in pursuit of information as well as contacts.

Although I shared the naturopath's suggestion with my doctors, they were unresponsive. I then embarked on securing a medical diagnosis as I was adamant that anxiety/depression was not going to remain on my records unquestioned. I was on my own, however. Fortunately I am no stranger to accessing information and I followed up every lead. I was eventually directed to a GP who treated ME patients privately and he made the diagnosis.

Winter

Aspen

The knife of illness
whittles my life
to harsh loss
sharply pruned
honed
to bare beauty
spirit tied
to a post
in the wind
my root
is growing
unseen.

I know winter,
its cruel ravishment
its hard seductive
numbing stare –
winter the portal
demanding payment
suspending life
stripping me
of greed

My choice is leaving
fear at the gates
healing seeds
enchanted growth
making possible
exultant songs
for spring.

Part Two

Family, Friends and Community

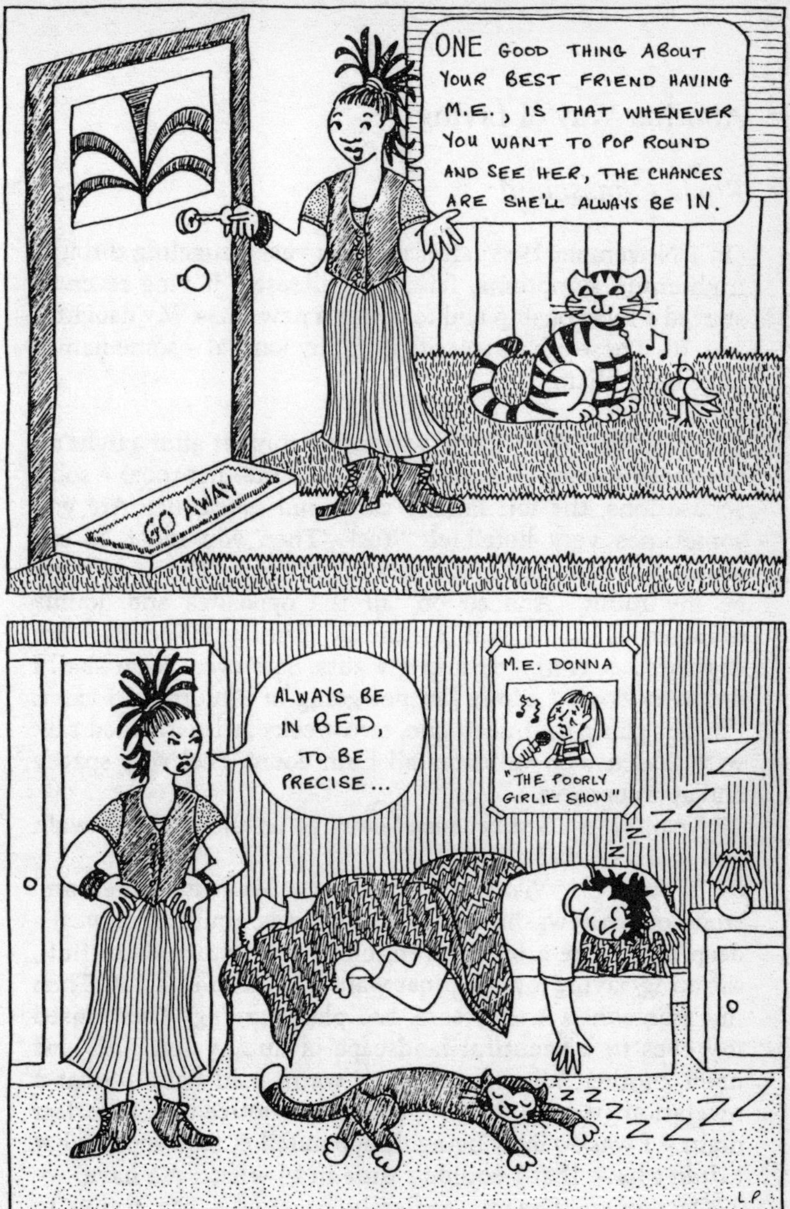
ONE GOOD THING ABOUT YOUR BEST FRIEND HAVING M.E., IS THAT WHENEVER YOU WANT TO POP ROUND AND SEE HER, THE CHANCES ARE SHE'LL ALWAYS BE IN.
GO AWAY
ALWAYS BE IN BED, TO BE PRECISE...
M.E. DONNA
"THE POORLY GIRLIE SHOW"
ZZZZ
ZZZZZZZ
L.P.

Another Way of Living

Rosie Chasseaud

On 1 November 1989, after nearly a year struggling through frightening symptoms, I finally collapsed, having recently started a relationship and teaching a new class. My daughter was 10. These are fragments from my journal – some names have been changed.

5 November 1989   Laura was lovely tonight after a fight all pm about sorting one box of stuff back into her room – sobs, accusations, the lot! Finally came and asked me: 'Are you sometimes very horrible?' 'Yes!' 'Then you must be my mum. Are you sometimes very nice?' 'Yes!' 'Then you must be my mum.' And so on, all the opposites and double negatives . . . a real synthesis. Brilliant! Feeling very depressed & grotty, pain in my guts. Sore eyes. What shall I do? Why don't I admit I'm not going in tomorrow? I can't. I'm not going to. I need one, two weeks at least. Good talk with Helen who validates all I am doing. Feel very spacey and apprehensive.

12 November   Sad because I can't go on the women's walk and it is a *beautiful* day.

27 November   Visions: sorting out a beautiful storeroom, stone or whitewashed clay, deep shelves, rounded curves, a deep place like a bread oven, clean but with rolls of fluff, thinking/saying joyfully, Just wait till I clean this out! Then my stomach: a small, sore, sad place, *crying*. Then raised my eyes to a beautiful landscape of humpy soft hills one upon another, all suffused with warm gold light – what a revelation: it was there but I hadn't noticed it. Like last night – I was so busy being disappointed & sore about what I *didn't* have that I couldn't tune in to what I did have.

3 December   Dream: endlessly packing a bag trying to

leave some unpleasant damp place where someone had already appropriated my bed anyway. Ineffectively sorting belongings, taking far too long, missing a train . . . on and on. Only 'nice' bit: entrance was through Edwige's kitchen, small, intense, beautiful coloured glass, perched on the edge of somewhere, reached by rickety wooden steps. Alternative: drop everything, just go, cut loose, dump my useless baggage. What was keeping me there anyway? Decided to start visualisation for pain in my side: feels more entrenched, sinister, less willing to come to light; reluctant to tackle it. On days like today when Helen & I are both unwell and distant (she didn't offer touches or kisses) I get scared, lose touch with times we have just had of intimacy, closeness, contentedness.

17 December   Can't sleep despite two sleepless nights of wind and rain. Don't understand. We've come away together, made love wonderfully, tenderly the first night but not since. Walking in the rainy woods today, sharing beauty, felt tender and erotic, wanted to lie down right there and make love on beds of leaves. I've offered lovemaking all day and she has evaded me, finally by going to sleep. She offers closeness but it doesn't feel enough. Hurt, disappointed, no, furious that my offering is rejected. As if I have to damp down my erotic side. She will tell me I ought to conserve my energy, I'm not looking after myself. Fuck that. I hate always being the 'problem' one.

10 January 1990   Feel unreal, depressed at the moment, ineffectual. Can't do anything, don't want to. Where has my energy gone? Rose pointed out last week's drugs [gastroscopy] won't have helped any. What is the matter with me? Suddenly feel I am making it all up. Whom can I trust if I can't trust myself?

16 February   My head feels open and vulnerable at the top, an open bag with a drawstring, not protected enough. Need a hard hat! Everything is flying away, can't focus.

24 February   Dream about Laura: sending her in small car down narrow steps, across road. At first okay but then in large car which she can't control. 'Put on the brakes!' She can't reach. Car careers up and down hill, people try to help, finally crashes, she is killed. I'm sending her out into something she can't handle – she's not grown-up enough yet. In dream I'm injured – people are lifting me around. So I should really be doing it but can't because I'm incapacitated.

8 March Trouble walking now – my legs don't work properly.

22 March Ache with weariness though guts better. Scared at my weakness: walking and climbing stairs leaves me breathless and faint. Can't believe this is happening to me.

15 April Hard week coming to terms with non-mobility, no longer being part of community, someone who makes things happen. A lot of things to mourn. Good moments with Laura, though also a bit rough – she learnt to make tea, cook scrambled egg on toast, hang washing: proved herself very competent!

24 April Today I feel a prisoner – ravaged by Helen's announcement that she's going abroad for a week. Says she often doesn't tell me what she's thinking – I already have enough on my plate!!! I said, 'Tell me! It hurts when you don't!'

18 May Tired, depressed. Doc. checked heart symptoms: numbness, faintness when I walk or get very upset. Heart okay. Feel a fraud. Lynne [therapist] asked, 'Can you think back to a time when you were well and full of energy?' I couldn't. Upset. Surely that can't be true? I must be misremembering.

31 May Heart thumping away waiting to be assessed for Mobility Allowance. Humiliating having to prove I'm 'disabled'.

9 June Must our relationship be like this? *So* hard, *so* painful? Can't bear the way the energy flows/stops/flows/stops. She's angry with me for the energy I use up. I'm angry and fed up with her. Feel very spaced out, out of control. Maybe it's the medicine. Can't stand not to be touched and held. She doesn't want to be with me when I have a sick headache. I'm exhausted with being tossed up and down. Helen does lots for me (special food, washing up, bedmaking) even when she's tired and pushed, and I'm not even grateful! (All I want is a hug!) I want more, yet more precious energy. I think she likes to do it – caring. But also feels it a duty and a burden. Will suggest she give up looking after me for now and we see what happens. Spend (even) less time together? Meanwhile I'll look elsewhere for my physical needs. Feel clear and strong about this now instead of stuck inside my despair and fury.

10 June Waking from vivid, terrifying dreams all week, sometimes with pounding heart.

11 June Sick headache, not made better knowing that Helen wouldn't want to see me like this.

13 June Sore chest: coughed up nasty phlegm. Can't settle to anything, feel numb, sore. If our evenings together are to be 'quality time' when do we sort out the shit? Or is she right – should we only have nice times together? What if I don't feel okay? Feels like a complete double bind to me.

15 June At concert last night closed my eyes, had visions of myself moving, dancing; realised how much I miss that.

17 June Feel funny having made decision about early retirement; cried on phone to [headteacher]. A break from teaching means leaving my school . . . my space, my 'home', my 'family' and all I've helped create. Head said he'd miss my creativity. Where do I put it now?

20 June Woke this night too with sweat pumping out of my chest! Eyes tired; sore, itchy chest. I ache.

21 June Helen said she wanted to 'stay apart' this weekend. Hell! Some people spend easy time together, some even live together! Reckons she's picking up on my pain at some level, needs to sidestep to protect herself. And of course she's not supposed to do that! She's supposed to stay there and catch me!

5 July Lynne: important for me to stay in touch with my skills – like unemployed people – draw them, write them, create support group. I'm lonely. I need and want people – get on the phone! Strong sense of being somewhere else with Helen, of summing her up to see how far she fills my needs. Felt bad thinking about it, selfish. Helen pointed out I'm not just on the receiving end, I get to give as well. My point is that I don't get the chance if she has to filter me, doesn't want my presence. Maybe I must put all this energy somewhere else for now – into planting my garden, for instance.

15 July   Am deciding to end this relationship – can't believe it. Phoned Ulla – need to hear someone say they care about me, as I cry and cry. So, end of the affair. Said I couldn't bear any longer the pain of Helen's distance.

17 July   Not nearly so brave today. £50 gift from parents at school means plants for the garden and lovely art/sewing materials. How I ache with all these goodbyes, and then how free I feel! Gulping Bach flower remedies like mad! Hours with *Old Cottage Garden Plants* and Vita Sackville-West sorting out what will grow in my dry soil.

28 July   It's as if Helen has everything she wants at the moment and I don't feel I do – blank, despairing. She phones me nearly every day to boast (her word) of the success of various expeditions etc., full to overflowing of creative energy, while I'm the opposite. Basically okay, just quiet, interested in my garden, but there's still a big gap. Helen doesn't seem to feel it at all, and I do and I mind and feel envious, spiteful, angry!

30 July   Maman goes away today, Ulla's away, Louise is away, Helen's going away, Rose is away, Laura's going away. Panic. Heavy session with Lynne: fear my mother (if I told her my feelings) would crumple and disappear and there would be no one there for me. 'Who would there be?' I asked. 'You,' she said.

5 August   Tired sore eyes from so much sun, so many sleepless nights, so much crying, reading. Inspired by May Sarton: *Journal of a Solitude*. Want to celebrate my present 'solitude'. Certainly different from ever before, alone but not abandoned. If I retreat it's to lick my wounds, howl, heal myself. I hurt sometimes but am still whole.

21 August   I *mind* that my illness has affected our relationship so that we've not done many things I'd have liked us to do. I mind that she can do them with other friends, not me.

3 September   Louise has sent a beautiful gardening book, an opera tape and a hug card. Says, 'I find your home a very spiritual place'!!! Also, 'The first thing [my son] said to me when I got home was, 'Is Rosy all right?' He cares about you deeply and so do I.'

11 September   Wrote to DES, doc, LEA to appeal against no-pension decision. Very tired, excruciating tender pain under my right arm, in right breast. Have ordered some beautiful notebooks. Will ask Ulla to bring some too. Could do with Ulla *right now*.

29 September   Michaelmas. Soft grey rainy morning. Collected plants from nursery: globe thistle, eryngium, achillea (soft salmony pink), aconite and alchemilla. They will enjoy the rain while waiting to be planted. This garden gives me such pleasure.

30 September   Weary, dreadful to wake up aching: neck, shoulders, arms, lower back. Even this hand today. Wish I could discover pattern. Laura's making gingerbread. Panic when she consulted me in the midst of my preparations. Said firmly, "I *can't* deal with two things at once.' 'Okay,' she said. And then it *was* okay, but had to truly focus hard on what I was doing.

19 October   So tired I even didn't want to see Lynne. Want to record that I'm enjoying art classes, putting on weight, feel happy, calmer about Helen, spent some lovely time with Rose, am passionately into plants and catalogues!

23 October   Feel as if I don't exist. Helen, Rose and Ilse are the only women who contact me.

31 October   A year since I stopped work. Still don't put art first. Trouble is, I want to see people. Very tired, shoulder hurts, stops me working.

1 November   Just had second bath to ease neck and shoulders. Organised deck chair in glasshouse for needlework – now have somewhere sunny to work – good! Slept pm. Woke aching and grotty.

2 November   Dismayed how much my course takes out of me; something has to change if I'm to get better. Too tired to do *anything* – just want to be looked after. Need to cut out housekeeping, socialising. Miss a class? Ouch. Must be ruthless.

1 December Laura's dressing up as a Roman empress in front of my mirror. She's tired and glandy, fed up with my being tired and unavailable. Has tiny breasts growing. My arm and shoulder have hurt like hell all week. Missed Monday's art class, left Thursday's early.

5 December Lying in bath images came of being trapped by stretchy web of greyish live stuff – my illness. I'm allowed to escape every so often but sooner or later have to lie down under it again.

12 December Drained, on edge, because of this pain. No escape.

30 December Amazing crisis: *pain* in shoulder/neck/back, left hip; sore throat, cold, long overdue period and diarrhoea! But went to bed with strange luxurious sense of okayness and actually slept. Still fragile, bellyachy, weepy, but fine. Making a list of things I want!

15 January 1991 Sleeping badly because of pain: everything hurts, even writing. Lynne suggested I pull in my resources, past/present/future: imagine walking holidays with Rose, summer garden, warmth, friendship, concern, help from various people. Past?? sense of landscapes/ achievements but all tainted by anxiety. How to salvage? Would make me more 'here', more solid.

5 February Seething with frustration and pent-up rage, want to scream, grind teeth, stamp, aargh! grrr! tremendous power. Dreams: trying to force issues. *Pain* in shoulder, arm, across chest – wants to burst out. Something wanting to get born. My only power at the moment: my art, ordering seeds, planting garden. Otherwise, *waiting* . . .

12 February Whole day just for me. Suddenly doing a lot more, art especially. Much pain still in right shoulder, numbness lying down, pins and needles both arms. Periods still up the creek. Sore belly, looseish bowels. Latest remedies for heart and circulation, usual liver and bio-stuff, also anti-antibiotics! Achievements of last six weeks: I've bought/given myself half of my list. Alan is doing mortgage for me. Have ordered veg seeds, reapplied for NHS and Community Charge exemptions, Income Support.

2 March   Oh but it's slow. Fed up with being ill, wondering if I'll ever get well . . . So many friends leaving: Rose going in August: who will be my best friend? A bit bleak, bereft. Who am I now?

9 March   Feel I'm remaking myself, and it's very lonely. Rose understands. At some level I know I'm going to be all right. And maybe having to be still is teaching me *how* to be still, centred, earthed – here, now, instead of yearning to be elsewhere. Learn contentment. Watch my garden grow. Draw myself! draw what is here – a lifetime!

27 March   Returned humiliated and angry from medical. Pottered in the garden, pruning bushes and things in the blazing sun. Whole day of bliss yesterday: went to Sissinghurst! I co-ordinated it all, including wheelchair. They took turns to bump me round. Most beautiful, hot, hazy day.

14 April   Fight with Laura about going to the shops. Had to threaten her before she would go. Not nice. When she won't do a 15-minute job like that I am really angry and desperate. Feel wounded now.

16 April   Still fearful, untrusting of my own creativity. Need lots of nurturing at the moment. Invited Margaret and Joyce for tea yesterday, chatted in the garden. Rose is the only one I can really talk to about it all: compassionate and supportive . . . talked about various challenges, illness, relationships . . . the people who respond are the ones who grow, become good friends – as she and I did.

30 April   Life is very busy (and nice) with Laura here full-time. Luckily had more energy lately but using it up fast. Ulla saying, 'I think of you daily!' I found very moving; relief – I can let go and just be myself.

30 June   Very depressed. Laura has gone for the day. Miserable that the house is so tatty and grimy and messy. Task for July: tidy, sort, clean, get friends to help.

17 July   Managed to do three studies from photos of Ulla's old blue-green doors – going to try some experiments on canvas.

22 July   Have very tired sore eyes with tics. So no reading, no art for a while . . .

29 July   Sad call from Laura at camp – promised I would go on Wed. Esther came for the evening, lovely chats, kisses, cuddles. I love the way she touches my neck, shoulders, arms, kisses my eyes.

11 August   Absolutely exhausted. Esther came and spent the day, she and Laura looked after me.

12 August   Laura thoroughly sad, weepy, negative, sorry for herself, and I thoroughly exasperated with her. Bought her school shoes, sandals, canvas shoes, took her for a haircut. Sometimes I feel so detached - it's quite freaky – no one exists, not Rose, not Ulla, not Louise – as if I just didn't care about them, nor they about me. That's when I think I'm mad – moving away from them, in another world where they simply don't impinge. Some parts of dying must be like this.

13 August   *Exhausted* today. No strength in arms even. In bed. Laura much better. Doc yesterday for sore bum and weight loss: nothing obviously wrong, took blood for thyroid test.

22 August   I've come down to the beach: my first walk out on my own like this for 18 months! This is what I need!!! Tide is in, sun is warm, breeze not too strong or cool. How strange to be coming to know a person who brings 40-odd years of experience with her – all those lives.

31 August   Can't sleep. Sore tum. Aching arms, shoulder from watering garden. Too many thoughts. Read Esther Irena Klepfisz's poem about the maiden aunts – want to say to her, 'Look – this is me, this is what I want to share with you, this energy, this celebration, this triumph.'

7 September   Ulla rang to say, 'How about a cup of tea?' Lovely!

15 September   Saw Dr K on Friday: says my immune system/gut has packed up again. Felt very upset, weepy. Got used to it a bit by now. Rose came yesterday, made tea, had long chat on my bed, about new things in Manchester she is looking forward to. Talked about my illness, over two years now, why I might have relapsed. Getting involved with

Esther was simply one factor . . . Symptoms now: leaden limbs, aching glands and lymph nodes, sore guts, 'indigestion'. Can hardly move. Just have to *stop* again & reflect & be. Let go of all hope & expectations. Start *again*.

18 September With Lynne yesterday looked at my fear of my illness, of never being okay again, of never feeling my creative/gardening energy again. She affirming that all my selves are one woman, not in fact separate selves. That I do not become unlovable by becoming ill.

21 September I hate that Esther is fearful because of my illness, yet she is and all we can do is live it and see.

2 October Totally unable to sleep though bone-aching with tiredness. Esther's fears of my illness – all feeds into my dread that it makes me bad and unlovable. God – this seesawing! Because at moments I can say/know/mean it: 'I am going to get well, I am alive and creative and wonderful. I am worth loving. I have much to offer, ill or not.' I *know* that life will win out but fear otherwise. I *will not* give in. *I refuse to die.* I find it so hard to believe in Esther's love when she is backing away from me in terror! Yet at times we are very open to each other, very close, very 'present'.

6 October One day at a time – that's all I can do. Esther says she loves me and all she can do now is to go back and start all over again. At the very least she wants a friendship . . . My strongest feeling is a despair and horror that I can never qualify because I am ill, thin, angry, in pain. I can do no magic thing to make me okay.

8 November Very quiet and still today, can hardly move. But it's good. Postcard from Rose – her letters keep me going. Plus sessions with Lynne. Margaret and Joyce came, recounted their adventures in France.

12 November Back into solitude . . . Yet I was happy on Sun, felt absolutely happy just being me. So, what is my life now? My daughter, my cats, my friends, garden . . . I've mended/finished a lot of things lately, a lot of unfinished business . . . Lynne asked me what I wanted and I said a relationship based on joy not pain.

24 December Card from Esther: 'I'm sorry that things did

not work out between us – it has not been an easy time for either of us.' Her first letter to me. Now maybe we can be friends.

27 December Dreams about my father. In one he was advising/ interfering about some artwork. I yelled so loudly I woke myself up! In another I had apparently planted the odd hyacinth or daffodil bulb in the corner of the kitchen where there was bare earth, and now they were coming up through the kitchen floor! Sounds nicely subversive to me!

31 December Remembering my bulb dream makes me smile. I am *alive*. No one can stop me – I am going to go on living and blooming and growing.

In 1995 my dear friend Ulla died of breast cancer. In 1996 Laura started Sixth Form College, I turned 50 and began the final project of the textile course I started seven years ago. I'm growing stronger every year.

Once I was Ill and Now I'm Not: The Story of a Child With ME

In the Words of Valerie and Abigail Wright, Mother and Daughter

Introduction: Caeia March

Several years ago, one of my lovely nieces, who is now almost 19, contracted a devastating childhood illness. The following tape transcript is from a telephone interview with my sister and my niece. We look back on that time and on my niece's recovery since that time. It ends with myself and my niece talking about how she is now. We have included this in the book because we feel that this 'case study' throws up important questions about how mothers and girl children are sometimes disbelieved in our society. It takes great strength for any family to deal with a chronically ill child. For the child herself there may be fear and confusion, alongside the physical suffering.

This story has a happy ending. Such cases exist in all of the literature of ME. Some sufferers can and do recover. For my niece's and her family's sake, I am glad that we can say, once she was ill and now she is not.

The transcripts:

Would you start by telling me how it all began, Val?

Well, it was the April when Abbey was nine, and she started to have sore throats. She had two lots of antibiotics for the sore throats and after that, she began to be lethargic. In the May she was tired all the time and not particularly wanting to go to school, though she *went* to school; but after school she didn't really want to do anything. The significant one was that she didn't want to go to Brownies – which she'd enjoyed up until that time.

From the July, as we went into the six weeks' summer holidays, we hadn't booked a holiday away but we were having one or two days out. And the first day out was planned for a seaside trip, and she seemed to enjoy that, but she had swum in the sea in Bridlington, and had a very high temperature and was 'off' with headaches, and just wanting to stay in bed for three or four days after that.

– *Did you think she'd caught something from the sea?*

– Yes. We wondered if she had. Yes. And then the following week we had a day trip on a train, stopping at Appleby, and we went in a café and she'd had a meal that included, I think it was a pasty, but it didn't seem to be particularly well cooked. And she was very 'off' after that, for three or four days. She had a high temperature and headaches. The headaches became the feature from then on – together with lethargy and muscle pain. She was having severe headaches and we were using quite a lot of paracetemol, which is what the GP had said to use for the headaches.

And when it came to the third week of the holidays, we were having a day trip to London, but she wasn't well enough to go. We had her back to the GP who thought that perhaps she'd had a viral illness, possibly glandular fever, and she had blood tests but they came back negative.

Then we just seemed to go from bad to worse. By the end of the six weeks' holiday, she didn't go back to school. Was too tired to go. Her muscles were aching and her joints were bad.

– *In what way were her joints bad?*

– Well, she complained about them, especially her knees. Pain. In her knees and in her shoulders. She didn't particularly want to get dressed in the morning. Would go all day just in night clothes. And just didn't get back to school.

The next thing was that she became very constipated. This went from bad to worse. The GP wasn't really very helpful. She said, 'Oh, give her some laxatives. Do stop wittering on, Mother.' She more or less threw a packet of glycerin suppositories at me and told me to get on with it. Which I did. The poor child was in a terrible state. She would go for days. She simply couldn't do a pooh. She was desperate.

So because she seemed to be going downhill, they said they'd take her into hospital for physical investigations for a weekend. It was a bit of a disaster.

– *In what way?*

– She was taken into hospital as a malingerer. If she didn't get off the bed to go to the trolley for anything to eat, she wasn't fed. And I appeared at something like half past ten, on the Saturday morning, with fruit and stuff, and she'd not had any breakfast. All the nurse would say was, 'Well, the breakfast came and went, but she didn't make the effort.'

– *Oh, Val . . .*

– She hadn't got off the bed to go to the trolley to get her Cornflakes or whatever, and of course they were treating her as being old enough to do that, at nine and a half. But she, you know, her body, she couldn't push it. At times, her legs seemed to not work. The hospital attitude was, 'We've got really ill people in here, you're wasting our time.' I think they were cruel. No one even came and talked to her. No one even asked her how she was. I think that they did a lot of damage. Psychological damage. We felt that it was an awful place. We couldn't wait to get her home. And I think she generally became very frightened that weekend. But from that weekend in hospital they suggested that we had to have family therapy.

We did go to one family therapy session – but we didn't take it up again. It meant bringing Belinda out of school – she was just newly into secondary school and I thought she had enough on, just starting secondary school and having a sister who was ill, apart from being labelled as part of a family that perhaps wasn't quite right. So we didn't pursue that, and that's when we had the psychologist sent to the house.

We weren't given a choice. And I didn't agree with the psychologist coming to the house, so I froze him out. I made sure he was cold while he was here. I didn't offer him a coffee, or put the fire on! He stopped coming.

– This was in the autumn?

– Yes. September/October time. But nothing seemed conclusive. We felt she had an illness of sorts but didn't know what it was. Putting it down to the aftermath of glandular fever, but we hadn't got a diagnosis. By now she was failing fast. Under the duvet, didn't want to come out. We felt it was a physical illness that was becoming psychological because she was by now very frightened indeed. Nobody could tell her what it was. The physical symptoms were moving into mental disorder. I think that was because no one was able to put a finger on it. Nobody really seemed to be helping.

– No name for it?

– No. That's right. And not particularly being believed. Such as, outpatient clinics were pretty poor on everything – 'We can't examine you unless you'll climb on the couch *yourself*', sort of thing. When she couldn't actually get on to the couch herself, nobody offered to help her. It was, 'No, Mother, you must leave her to do it herself.' They were suggesting that *we* weren't being particularly helpful. That *we* were making her ill. It was the suggestion that it was coming from us, which was quite uncomfortable. But we knew that this lethargy had gone on from the Easter-time. By now she had severe muscle weakness. It was becoming a psychological illness because nobody was able to sort out the physical illness.

I floated between thinking this child is ill and then, well, this child could be making more effort. It was a bit of both with me really at that time. So I used to push her quite hard. I'd make her come out of the house. Rightly or wrongly. I'd make sure she did some physical activity most days.

The distances she could walk would be either round to the library, or to a friend's house. I would make sure she'd done that. She didn't want to. I think, looking back, that my idea was, things seize up if you don't use them. With joints it's a balance between rest and activity. I thought that some activity for a child was going to be better than the rest. We'd had a physiotherapist come to the house who was very intent on her moving her joints. I think that's probably why I got the idea that, yes, this is a good thing. Because you mustn't have muscles shortening in a child of that age. She was still in her growth years. And I remembered the old idea from the polio victims, that you must massage the muscles, must keep them going.

– *So at what point did you start the swimming?*

– Quite late. We didn't discover warm water until the November. I just suddenly thought, she needs to move, and probably moving in water might be easier for her. So in November I took her down to a baby pool I thought might be open and when it wasn't, the attendant was very helpful and kind to us. He told us about a swimming bath that was warm because it was designed for the polio victims of the past, and nowadays used as a swimming club for anyone disabled. Arthritis evenings, polio evenings, goodness knows what. So the water was kept a higher temperature and the changing rooms were all hot. There were ramps down into this pool. It was an old-fashioned pool that had been converted. You paid ordinary council swimming rates for it. I took her twice a week. She didn't have to go down steps or over the side into deep water. She could just walk very slowly down the ramp into it. She could go in as if going off a beach.

We didn't have hotels with sports clubs then like they do now. There weren't a lot of facilities. It's going back a bit, isn't it? And we didn't have much money in the family. I mean, I daren't give up my job, two mornings and two evenings a week. I was a nurse in family planning at the time. Various clinics.

– How did you manage with childcare that autumn?

– Betty. She's my Godmother. She came with her car and picked Abbey up, wrapped her in blankets, took her out. She'd do that for the mornings I worked.

–Did Abbey look forward to that?

– No. Not always. Each day was different. She could wake up fine; she could wake up very low. It would depend what sort of night she'd had. She had bad nights sometimes because she had bad headaches. I mean, we never exceeded the amount of paracetemol that a child should have but she was often up to the limit. I was given the guidelines that it was better to make sure she had the paracetemol every four hours rather than let the headaches come back. So, eventually we got into giving it her as a routine. She had that for weeks and weeks. Meanwhile the GP had diagnosed her as having depression, probably back in October-time. Abbey just couldn't get out of bed one morning. I called the GP, who came after morning surgery. She said, 'There's nothing wrong with this child apart from her being depressed.' She prescribed Amytriptyline to help her over her depression. But I didn't give it. I didn't agree with it. I decided I wasn't going to have her drugged up to the nines. I was quite upset. I thought, if she's depressed then there's a *reason*. The *reason* is that she believes she's desperately ill.

– Do you think that Abbey thought that she was dying?

– I think she probably did. Whether she would put that into words now, I honestly don't know. But, yes, I think she thought she'd got something very serious.

Meanwhile we had relatives who would peer at her and comment that she was terribly ill and wasn't anybody doing anything for her, which didn't help; and we had neighbours who thought that we were the problem – that we'd somehow as a family unit, caused it.

– So, at some point Abbey went back to school, did she?

– She started back to school part-time late November. The teachers were sending work home, and they suggested to us that they'd take her, whatever she could manage. We'd take her some weeks in the mornings, some weeks in the afternoons. Some weeks she'd go two days. It was the swimming term and they thought that might be good for her, so they gave her extra time, to get on to the coach and off again the other end and so on. They were excellent. She was extremely slow. One or two of her friends were very helpful. She missed out on friends, because of the illness. There was one child who befriended her because this particular child hadn't any friends. Abbey realised she was doing this child a favour – and it didn't disturb her. She didn't mind. They became useful to each other.

Her other friends were kind but she'd been missing for quite a long time, and friends find other friends.

– What happened next?

– Well, she was very good at art, and she went in for the Halifax Building Society competition, and she won a prize. So she had to go up out of her seat in assembly to receive this prize. It took her an age. She walked so slowly. I think that highlighted how bad she was. I don't think she realised. She was just so used to being as slow as this. I don't think it was traumatic for her. She got an Oxford Dictionary and a ruler and a nice book, or something. She was going up to receive it. Thrilled to bits. She was helped to go up and get it.

It was after that assembly that one of the teachers saw me in Tesco's. We were in getting some bits for Christmas. This female teacher came up to me, she said, 'I think I know what's the matter with your daughter. I've read quite a lot about ME recently, and I'm pretty sure that that is classic for your daughter.'

– How did you feel when she said that?

– I'd thought this myself. And it was, sort of, someone

recognising, without me having to say, 'Well, I think she does have this problem.' So I was quite pleased that someone else was able to say to me, 'I think I understand that that's what's happening.' Because a lot of local people hadn't and some were very shocked by her appearance, if they hadn't seen her for a while.

– What did she look like?

– Her face was swollen, as if she was on steroids. I didn't realise how bad it looked until she'd had her school photo. I never kept it. I ripped it up because I was so upset by it. But I wish I'd kept it now. Her shoulders were hunched, and her head had gone down into her shoulders. She looked an ill child.

– She was an ill child.

– Yes, and the shoulder hunching, of course, was pain. Pain in her joints. So her shoulders had gone up and her head had gone down. So she had no neck. On the photograph she just didn't have a neck.

– So what happened slowly over the next year then?

– By the following Easter when she was ten, we had a party for her. She could invite whoever she wanted and we had it round at the local Methodist Hall. We had games and stuff and she thoroughly enjoyed that. Enjoyed the attention. Again we took one or two photos, and she still didn't look completely right. She hadn't grown. She was still the same size as the previous year and the amazing thing was, then, between ten and eleven all of a sudden she just shot up. She gained several inches in a year. That was very noticeable. Neighbours were saying, 'She's growing in front of us.'

– Like boys sometimes do?

– That's right, because she hadn't grown for a year. She'd been completely stunted.

– *What happened to the headaches?*

– They just gradually went. We just noticed that we were giving her less paracetemol. So the headaches went but the tiredness didn't. She remained tired. After *any* event. For a long while. She was in her third year junior when she was ill, then luckily she had one more year before she moved to secondary, or else I don't think she would have managed the move. She would've been too tired to travel. But luckily, she gradually improved. Enough to be able to do mostly what everyone else was doing. She helped herself along by learning to manage it. Like at the swimming baths she'd pretend she'd done a length when she hadn't. She hid under the water and waited for the others to swim back then bobbed up and joined them again. Things like that! (Laughter) She got round it. In lots of different ways.

– *So she sort of learnt to manage it?*

– Yes. That's right. She learnt to manage it. She learnt to become unnoticeable. You know, to fade in with everyone.

– *So how did the tiredness affect the transition to secondary school?*

– It did affect it. There were things she couldn't manage on the sports side. That became quite marked in the first term at secondary school. There was an open evening and I let them know at school that she'd had a post-viral illness and that her stamina wasn't what it might be and that some of the sports she wouldn't manage. I said, 'If she can't do something, I'm sorry, but she won't be having you on, she actually physically can't do it. And I'd prefer it if you wouldn't push it or she'd have to have that session at home.' I made that quite clear. They were kind and we didn't have any problems.

– *How was she in the evenings?*

– She didn't join any clubs or after-school activities at all.

She seemed to already know how to manage the tiredness. But she did go to things locally. She went to a local youth club. She enjoyed doing that with local friends because they didn't go to the same school and that was how she got to see them. She went to Guides as well. If she was all right she did the things and if tired she stayed home. No one ever pushed her. That went on for three years.

– So by then her body had a sense of what she needed to do?

– Very much so. In the morning, if I went to wake her up for school and she was either unrouseable or she said 'I don't feel well this morning,' then she had the morning off. She'd go in at lunchtime. I'd ring the school and say, 'My daughter's woken with a sore throat,' something physical I'd put on it, 'and if she's better later she'll be in.' So that she wasn't marked absent.

– So you'd ring up?

– Oh, yes, fairly regularly. Probably about once a week. All that first year at secondary school she'd have one morning off. My attitude was, well, school work will get done, if she's well enough, and it doesn't if she's not.

– And did you have in your mind at that time that the teacher who had seen you in Tesco's was actually right and this child had ME?

– Yes. We didn't know a lot about it. I knew she'd had a post-viral illness. That's what I would have called it at that phase. We knew even then, even ten years ago, that if somebody had had bad flu they could be weeks and weeks getting over it. So she'd had something similar and it was taking that bit longer because it had taken a turn for the worse.

– So even had you not called it ME, you would have known that it was post-viral fatigue?

– Oh, yes. I was well aware of teenagers having glandular fever and sometimes not being right for a year. I thought that she must have had glandular fever, even though it was coming up negative. So this was the aftermath of that. Nobody'd said she'd got a brain tumor or anything like that, so we presumed that eventually she would come right. And she did.

– *Do you think that it affected her with her studying for GCSE?*

– Now then, I don't know which way round this is. She got through her GCSEs without a bat of an eyelid. She got ten. I think she then thought the academic scene was going to be totally easy. And got a terrific shock first year in 'A' level. But that might be nothing to do with post-viral illness. That might be personality. Because that happens to quite a lot of clever teenagers. But I do think the self-belief bit has always been a bit difficult. Your self-esteem is lowered if you think that after a night on the tiles you're laid out whereas everybody else can keep going. I think you begin to sort of not believe you can do things. I think she lost a lot of confidence and has never really thought of herself as being clever.

I think, you know, she *is* clever, and that's been a good thing. Because if she'd been a borderline reader, or had learning problems, then she'd have been wiped out with this. Probably never to recover. But once the headaches started to fade, and she could get back to reading, even though she wasn't physically able to do an awful lot, so long as she could read she was away, because she'd always loved reading. As she was sitting in the chair, I just kept supplying her with the stuff. She may not have gone to school but she would go round the library, sit for an afternoon there while I did my shopping, and the librarian was wonderful with her. She got into all the story tapes. So a lot of the classic tales that she probably wouldn't have read, she'd heard on tape.

So it was the librarian and the class teacher who were wonderful to Abbey. Not the one who saw me and said I think your daughter's got ME. No, her class teacher was a male teacher and I couldn't have faulted him. He encouraged her over what she *could* do. He'd say, 'While they are doing that would you like to do this?' So she was supplied with stuff to do the whole time and stimulated. They were the two who were very, very helpful.

– *Do you think that there is anything now that Abbey is affected by? Any legacy?*

– Concentration and memory. Her concentration span is short and her memory she struggles with, and I think that's why she probably didn't do as well as she might have done with her history 'A' level. She chose a subject where she needed to have a good memory and it failed her at times. But that may not be the ME. Who knows? She may not *have* a good memory.

– *What about general social activities? Does she still get a bit tired at times?*

– She burns the candle at both ends! She's a very active person. She's out a lot. Has a lot of friends. She's very sociable. And expects everything to just happen. She's not too hot on organisational skills. (Laughter)

– *You mean* ME *intersecting with personality?*

– Yes. (Laughter)

– *D'you think she's made a more or less full recovery?*

– I think so. But I don't know. Because I don't know if memory is part of it. And the memory did let her down quite badly at times doing the 'A' levels and it caused a reasonable amount of frustration.
– *I can't think of anything else I need to ask, Val. Is there anything else you want to add?*

– No, thanks, love. Abbey is here. I'll just go and get her.

– *Thanks. And thanks, Val, for the interview.* [Pause] *Hi, Abbey, how are you?*

– I'm all right, thanks. How are you?

– *Oh fine, thanks. You know Val and I have been taping this thing about when you were little and you had your illness? I wondered if you'd talk to me about any of the things you can remember about it, things you want to say?*

– Yes, I will, but I don't really remember that much.

– *I wondered about that. D'you think you've blocked it?*

– I think I did actually. I remember very little. I do remember that when I got to secondary school, I was always tired still. I was always run-down and I knew I'd had a viral thing. I still get tired sometimes but I don't remember a great deal. I still have symptoms that come to the surface now and again, but I really don't remember much.

– *That's probably a good thing. Do you think it affects you now? Are there moments when you think, oh, that's the tiredness come back?*

– Yes I do. If I have a series of late nights, all the others can cope with it but I get quite run-down and I get colds easily. Now and then I get very, very tired.

– *Is there anything you do about that? Do you just battle on or do you give yourself half a day in bed, or something?*

– (Laughter) Oh, I'm quite often asleep. (We both laughed.) I don't take days off work or anything. It doesn't happen very often now, because I try not to get too tired.

– *I'm glad you're through the other end of it now. Obviously, it's marvellous to be looking back on it. Rather than looking forward and thinking uggggh, you know? (We both laughed.) I want to put it in the book, Abbey, because it's a recovery story and I think it'll be encouraging for other young women who maybe have got it or aren't as far on in their recovery. Have you ever met any other young women who had anything similar?*

– I don't think I know anyone. Something rings a bell but I can't think who. It was a long time ago.

– *Yes, it was. A very long time ago. Do you remember any of the swimming incidents?*

– I do remember the time at juniors, in our last year, when we all had to do our eighteen lengths. I was an hour longer than everyone else. They all had to wait for me. Everyone else had got out and I still had eight lengths to go.

– *I'm amazed you could even manage it.*

– I shouldn't have tried it at all. I was absolutely exhausted. Like one of those frustration dreams.

– *What, when your legs are going and nothing's getting any nearer?*

– Yes. It was awful.

– *What about other times since then? Do you think it affected 'A' levels at all?*

– I don't know. I know I didn't have as much stamina as other people. We were all working quite hard. I used to get run-down then and felt very tired. I know that my memory's very bad. I don't know if that's anything to do with it, but I'm terrible at remembering things.

– *It's one of the classic symptoms. Those of us who are now approaching menopause have a giggle about it. Because it's one of the symptoms of menopause as well, so if one doesn't get you the other one will. (We both laughed.) I rang this woman for the* ME *book and I said, 'I'm really sorry I've forgotten to phone you,' and she said, 'Don't worry, we had this conversation last week.' (Much laughter.) Do you find your memory is worse if you are very tired?*

– Oh, yes. I get very confused when I'm tired. I'll talk a load of gibberish to people, not realising things.

– Do you lose words, and bits of sentences?

– Oh, yes. I lose the ends of words.

– Even now?

– Oh yes. But only when I'm very tired. I'm really not affected for a long time if I get enough rest.

– And you've learned to manage it so that you get your rest, have you?

– Oh yes. I mean, it doesn't bother me at all. I get tired, but so do a lot of people, and my memory is bad but it might have been anyway.

– You mean that might just be you and not the ME?

– Yes. I mean, I might just be an absent-minded fool! (Much laughter.)

– Is there anything else you can think of about that childhood illness that you want to add?

– Nothing else I can think of. How I see it is that I seemed to get better quite quickly. Maybe it wasn't like that, but from my childhood perspective it seemed to be over quite soon. Then it'd maybe come back again in relapses from time to time. Feeling tired. And that's all it's ever been, ever since. Not like a long awful convalescence. More like a steady recovery.

– With occasional bouts of extreme tiredness?

– Yes, but it's hardly, hardly happening. It's a normal life – well, it's normal for me, I just have a couple of extra hours in bed now and again. When I was a child I was ill and now I'm not. So, it helps to put a gloss on it. Once I was ill and now I'm not. And it's true.

– It's not really stopping you doing anything, is it? Your job, anything?

– No, and I'm going to have a very demanding job.

– *And with pots and pots and pots of money!*

– That'd be nice. (Laughter) I'd like to have my own business. I don't know how I decided I really want to get into antiques. But it *is* what I really want to do. I don't know where it came from. I've been really lucky getting this job as well. Loads of people write in for jobs at the auctioneers all the time.

– *Well if anybody asks, an auctioneer, why her? I say, because she's the right person for the job! Loves art, very sociable, and clever.*

– I don't know about that but they say I work hard and they're pleased.

– *That means you'll get a very good reference.*

–Yes, they said they would. I don't know when I'll hear if I've got a place on one of the courses. But I'll apply again next year if I don't get in.

– Good luck. And thanks, Abbey.

Notes
Information on good practice, education, and home tuition for children and young people can be obtained from Action for ME. There are youth groups, networks and penpal arrangements for support and friendship. See Resources List, Part One.

ME and Pregnancy

Sue Sholl

Personal Story

I have had two babies whilst suffering from ME. In 1983 I became pregnant with my first baby. It was *during* that first pregnancy that I contracted ME.

At six weeks pregnant I was a bit tired but nothing extreme. I also had non-stop nausea, morning, noon and night. At that time I was riding a bike to work, approximately two miles, some of it uphill. I cannot say exactly when things changed but it was literally overnight. I was working full-time as a receptionist, and one day at work I went to walk down the corridor and my legs just wouldn't work properly. Suddenly it became impossible to ride the bike home, my legs just became like lead. A rash appeared on my upper body; I checked with the midwife as I was worried about German measles. I was extremely tired, extremely cold, and I had a constant thirst which was checked for diabetes. Allergies appeared: I'd been wearing clip-on earrings for years then suddenly I couldn't wear them any more. I had trouble sleeping, lots of leg pain, restlessness and nightmares. I also started to get memory problems. It was *very* sudden, and it was when I was less than three months pregnant. I went to the doctor and asked if I could have my iron pills early because I was so tired. I told him about the leg pain and he suggested support tights; I tried them but it only made it worse. I now had to get a bus to work, but even that was difficult because I had pain standing waiting for it.

I suffered with cramp and was prescribed calcium and vitamin D tablets. I had immense difficulty staying awake, and sometimes I managed a rest at lunchtime, in the sick room, as the sister at work was very nice. I was sent home from work with migraines, and every evening I slept. I lost interest in the job I had loved. I managed to continue working up to Christmas: the baby was due in March. Once I finished work the problems remained but eased a bit now I was able to rest.

The labour was textbook; everything happened just as it should. For pain relief, once my waters had gone and the contractions were stronger I had gas and air. I requested this because I didn't want pethidine and I didn't want an epidural, though I'm not sure why. I felt gas and air was right for me. Despite a very long second stage I wasn't exhausted, they had to make a cut and then the baby was born.

Everything up until then had been put down to the pregnancy. I expected it all to disappear once the baby was born and of course it didn't. I breastfed for three weeks but it didn't go well and she went on the bottle. The baby didn't sleep well; in fact we both used to drop from exhaustion. I rested the baby on the arm of the settee when feeding her to save my arms. I did her bottles in the morning when I was at my best. I changed her on the floor with my legs out in front of me.

I kept two changing bags and later on two potties one upstairs and one downstairs. Unfortunately the baby didn't sleep well for two years and I had by now decided that maybe they were right, maybe it was down to the pregnancy. When she did start sleeping and I was getting a full night's sleep regularly and I was *still* tired, I went back to the doctor but I didn't get any answers. It took *seven years* to get a diagnosis. By that time I'd had my second baby (five years after the first).

In that second pregnancy, for the first six months it felt like I had legs again – there was a vast improvement. I kept getting viruses so my general health wasn't brilliant but my legs were. At six months I went downhill in a week, I don't know why: perhaps I increased my level of activity too much. I was now ten times worse than I had been and I never recovered from this. It was now difficult, at times, to walk at all and I had to give up my part-time job.

The labour with my second baby was very different. I started having contractions (very mild) six weeks before the baby was due. They continued on and off for the six weeks, becoming more frequent and stronger as time went on. Three days before the baby was due they were constant but irregular. They were strong enough to break my waters and I went into hospital at this time. They didn't have room on the labour ward so I was put on the ante-natal ward. My labour in total lasted three days. Forty hours of that was full-blown contractions. I had no pain relief in all this time. I wanted to get through it if I could without pain relief because I knew I reacted badly to drugs. By using position and the breathing I was taught at Parentcraft classes and the right mental attitude I got through it. Finally they took me to the delivery room to induce me. The doctor who examined me was amazed to find I was fully dilated. Something was stopping the baby being born so they set up a drip. Thirty-five minutes later she was born. The cord had been wrapped *four* times round her neck so this may have been the reason. I wasn't tired despite those forty hours of labour: your body seems to give you extra energy at this time, and this applied to both births. The baby was fine, I didn't have any stitches this time, and I felt on top of the world.

I was lucky: the baby slept well and was very placid. I breastfed for three weeks but found I didn't have enough milk so she went on the bottle. I manoeuvred things my way this time. I gave her bottles at room temperature, let her get herself off to sleep and woke her before I went to bed. I kept her by the side of me, bottle ready, and put an extra large nappy on at night which was left until morning. We both got a good night's sleep.

When I had the first baby to care for I would say my ME was mild. With the second I would say I was in the moderate category. There were lots of problems: fatigue, mobility and relapses. It is just a question of finding a way round them. For the fatigue I slept when she slept. For mobility problems

I used her buggy as a kind of mobile walking aid when I needed to. Once she was mobile, I kept her in the same room as me to save energy. I put the baby bath inside the big one so I didn't have to try and lift it and did her bath at my best time – mornings. The most difficult time was when I was in relapse. I would lie on the settee and do relaxation while she played or watched a video when she was older. The very worst time is when you are ill and they are ill. I would then do only the basics. I had help sometimes, from my husband, family and friends. When that wasn't possible I managed one way or another. My greatest source of help was Donna, my first baby. She understood the problems so well because she literally grew up with my having ME. I encouraged both of them to be independent as soon as possible, to make a sandwich and drink for themselves, that kind of thing. I explained about ME; even Jade when she was quite small could understand and adapt when things were explained to her. Once the children got to school age it became easier. Sometimes it was very difficult but the good far outweighed the bad. I wouldn't have missed it for the world.

Research

There has been very little research done on ME, pregnancy, childbirth and the offspring. For this reason there has been very little information available to date. A very small survey was done by one of the national ME organisations. Some research was done in Australia, and the process of gathering information has started in this country. There needs to be a great deal more done before a clear and comprehensive view can be given. The general findings to date seem to be:

PREGNANCY
A small number of pregnancies do not progress normally but this is the case in the general population and may or may not be due to ME. It seems to be more likely if the mother is in the early stage of ME with signs that suggest an active viral infection. The majority do proceed normally and although it

is impossible to predict the outcome for any individual case, the majority of women find that their ME symptoms improve during pregnancy. Some do relapse later in the pregnancy, and ME symptoms are likely to return in force after the birth at some stage. It is a *temporary* reprieve. It is thought that partial suppression of the immune system is the reason for the improvement (which occurs naturally in order to avoid rejection of the foetus – it is half of someone else's genes so could be taken as 'foreign' to the immune system). Some women feel their condition is unchanged by pregnancy; a small number feel worse. The advice is the same – get plenty of rest during pregnancy.

Once the decision has been made to have a child there is also the question of fertility. Difficulty getting pregnant could be due to ME or it could be that a baby has been put 'on hold' and as the woman's age increases fertility is lowered. Cost too can be a factor. If because of ME the woman (or man) is unable to work, can they afford a child? If they go ahead and the health of the ME sufferer deteriorates, the partner might have to give up work to care for them. The fluctuating nature of ME is perhaps one of the biggest worries. Who is going to take over during a relapse? Are there others around – family or friends who could take over at short notice? Is there any chance of help from outside agencies or even paid help? There are a great number of issues to consider but in the end it has to be a personal decision.

CHILDBIRTH

From the information to date it seems that *anything* can happen, from having a completely normal labour and birth to having problems. If there are going to be problems they are likely to be: contractions starting early, irregular contractions, a reaction to some forms of pain relief, and exhaustion during the second stage of labour (pushing the baby out). The advice that has been given is to learn as much as possible about childbirth, about different positions that might help in labour, about the different forms of pain relief, and to learn relaxation from Parentcraft classes. Another suggestion is to write out your ME symptoms, emphasising the muscle fatiguability, and perhaps to draw up a 'birth plan' – what you would ideally like to happen and what you would prefer to avoid. For example, you might prefer to try a less intrusive type of pain relief first, such as gas and air, but be willing to change this if circumstances dictate. If it is needed you have it at the ready rather than trying to explain at the time. Some women ask for a Caesarian in advance. It depends on the individual doctor whether they will agree to this and it means a general anaesthetic or an epidural (some women may react badly to these some might not). Some women feel that an epidural would be best because of the energy needed to cope with the pain. Still others are wary of drugs and fear a reaction to the drugs more than the pain. It may be best to keep an open mind and see how it goes.

BREASTFEEDING
This is a source of controversy. On the plus side it is said that breastfeeding is a great saver of energy (no bottles to be sterilised and made up). It is also a way that the baby will receive antibodies to infection. It is a good source of GLA (an essential fatty acid), a deficiency of which leads to allergies. Also, a totally breastfed baby does not need to be changed in the middle of the night as there is no ammonia present in the urine. Breastfeeding also appears to delay the onset of ME symptoms. On the minus side some women feel that it takes most of the body's energy to produce breast milk, so you may need to rest almost constantly to keep up the supply. Another disadvantage is that no one else can take over as they can with a bottle. Bottlefed babies tend to go longer between feeds and you know how much they are taking.

In the end it is a personal decision and perhaps, as with labour, it might be best to keep an open mind and if you want to try it – fine. If, for any reason, it doesn't work out there is always the option of the bottle. From the research done to date it appears that some women breastfeed their babies without problems, some do have problems, such as not enough milk. Perhaps the best news from the research to date is that all of the babies born to mothers with ME have been healthy in terms of ME: none so far have developed ME themselves.

Issues

It can be a very difficult decision whether to have a baby or not whilst suffering from ME. Many women wait several years in the hope of recovery or at least improvement, and for the illness to stabilise.

There are so many issues surrounding this subject. What most women want to know is if they will be able to cope with the extra demands placed on their body by pregnancy, childbirth and raising a child. How will pregnancy affect their ME? Will there be extra problems in labour? Should they breast or bottlefeed? Can they cope with the twenty-four hour, three hundred and sixty-five days a year caring, for maybe twenty years or more? Perhaps the most important question of all is, will ME affect the health of the child?

Some women may already have had the illness for many years and if they are in their late thirties and want children they may feel that time is running out. It can be a case of 'now or never'. There can be a partner's needs to consider. If their partner desperately wants children and is going to be supportive, can they deny them a family? If it's a man who has ME he may be just as unsure and in need of information. Half of the baby will be from his genes – can he pass anything on? Can he deny his partner a longed-for family? If a woman falls pregnant accidentally she then has to decide whether to go ahead with the pregnancy.

ME can mean so much loss – health, careers, interests and hobbies, a social life. Does it mean losing the chance of a family too?

There are so many questions and so few answers. Many women have asked their GPs and consultants for their view. Most have no answers. Without information and research findings to go on, what can their doctors tell them? Even if they are given advice it can often be confused: 'You've got years yet', 'Wait until you are better', 'You'll never cope', 'Go ahead, it will make you feel better'. Even the national ME organisations can only give general advice without any definite answers. The consensus of opinion seems to be that it is best to wait until the illness has stabilised and there are no signs that suggest an active viral infection (low-grade fevers, diarrhoea, tender lymph glands and throat infections). They also point out that there is a *possible* genetic susceptibility to ME. At this point in time no one knows whether this is the case or not. Other advice is to make sure the mum-to-be gets plenty of rest during pregnancy and has help available. Knowing how to 'manage' the illness would also be of great benefit. Some individual doctors admit their ignorance but are willing to be supportive. Some advise against it. Still others feel that the joy of a new child may well outweigh all the problems.

Some Further Comments on Pregnancy and Motherhood for Women with ME: Editor's Note

The decision whether or not to get pregnant and bring up a child entered into the lives of many 'out' lesbians in the 1980s. So, when Sue Sholl and I were discussing the writing of this article, she kindly agreed to leave a space for me here so that I could outline some of the issues that are being considered by lesbians who are in the process of raising offspring or deciding to have a baby.

There are so many alternative types of lesbian family. They can include mothers who have had children from before coming out as lesbians and who don't want any more children; single lesbians who enter into co-parenting arrangements with partners or friends; new couples who have settled down together and then decided that one of them would have a child to be raised by them both together; an older woman with grown-up children who settles with a younger woman who wants a child; two friends sharing a house, both being lesbians but not in a relationship, and one wants a child, which they will raise together; and a case I have known of a single lesbian who successfully decided to have a child and to raise it in a single-parent lesbian family. This woman was able-bodied and financially independent, in a good, well-paid job. She had an interested and supportive network of lesbian friends – the baby had so many godmothers I was quite envious!

The intense feeling of wanting a child will not simply go away because a woman has ME. I identify with Sue's descriptions of the process of wanting to get pregnant, wanting a child. Many women reading this will also identify with this. It is a central question in the lives of many women. So why should either the fact of ME, in a woman's life, or the reality of lesbianism, be an obstacle to her being a good mother? There is no one way to be a good mother – and it is important that, as mothers, we keep on saying this.

However, the decision to have a baby is a complex one for lesbians, the more so if the birth mother or co-parent/partner has ME. The same would apply to some other chronic illnesses and some disabilities too – if there is need for physical care or if excessive tiredness is involved.

Firstly – getting pregnant. For many years, lesbians have used artificial insemination by donor, in conjunction with ovulation predictors, to get pregnant – or, less frequently, they 'do it once' with a male partner, the traditional way! Both of these methods can also be used used by heterosexual women with ME, for whom frequency of lovemaking could be exhausting.

Secondly – managing fatigue. As Sue points out in her article, during pregnancy and after childbirth, rest is essential and women try to avoid relapse. It is this question to which I now turn. The fear of relapse is a fact of life for many women with ME. Obviously, the decision to get pregnant and raise a child will take into account how much support might be available from partners and from friends, whatever our sexual orientation. But what if society's negativity towards lesbian mothers amplifies this – and puts the whole parenting possibility at risk?

To safeguard the lesbian family – and for protection against outside interference – some lesbian parents and parents-to-be are now taking seriously the whole issue of who the legal carers are if the birth mother becomes chronically ill before, during or after pregnancy.

Lesbian parents-to-be may now enter into legal arrangements known as 'residency orders', which have a precedent in both English and Scottish law. Such an arrangement ensures that if one of the partners becomes seriously ill or disabled the other has recognised rights and responsibilities in the law for the care of the baby/children. This means that the baby's carers – the two women – are named under the law, so that the baby does not have to undergo the trauma of losing either of its mums if a dispute arises in the wider world as to who is now 'responsible for looking after the baby'.

The residency orders also have other uses (in the unfortunate event of the lesbian family breaking up), but here I am describing them as they relate to illness and disability. ME is quite enough of a nightmare in any family, so for lesbian parents – including those who are considering having a child – it is important to avoid the risk of the baby/children being removed or claimed, against the wishes of its lesbian parents. In most areas Lesbian Line can give women the relevant numbers for legal advice. If in doubt, phone Lesbian Line London – they have the numbers for the rest of the country (see Resources List).

Love's a Funny Thing

Liz Tucker

Love's a funny thing, that's what I remember thinking. It makes you all floppy and tired, no concentration, no appetite. All your get-up-and-go just gets up and buggers off. Well, the Love of Your Life only comes along once in a lifetime, if you take any notice of Babs Cartland, so how do you know how it's going to feel?

Three months later, I was bedridden with glandular fever. My Love was still around, but long gone were my beloved business, income and merry little active life!

That was three years ago. Now there's the first faint glimmer of a possible longed-for return. Over those years there has been plenty of time to point the finger of blame – at me, of course. If only I had been able to read the signs earlier – but what signs were there?

Perhaps I had been overdoing it a little bit more than usual, but I didn't get into the office till gone five in the morning and was always home by, say, midnight, that's if I didn't have to work through. And I only drove about 10,000 miles a month, and I always had Sunday afternoon off. Usually, anyway.

But this was no problem. I had oodles of energy and if I had gone home at six I'd have been fidgeting about annoying the cats and wondering why I'd bothered paying for a TV licence. An evening's entertainment consisted of regional news; everything I could ever want to know about boats, dog mess and tripping over a kerbstone; or a sitcom, featuring everything but humour; or a tough cop show whose tough cop gets constant grief from his boss and a token woman, and which always starts at nine o'clock.

Things started to go astray when I met My Life, man of my dreams. I just couldn't keep my mind on the job, so to speak. Felt tired and had the odd dizzy spell. All quite above board for a lovestruck girlie. Then once mister wonderful was fully installed in living sinfully, I just woke up one morning and couldn't go any further.

Zombification. I think I invented that word. I watched those old horror movies and saw myself as one of those pale dummies with blank expressions, except they seemed fortunate enough to be able to move about unaided.

The illness resembled a magpie in my nest. I didn't want it there and there was no way of getting rid of it, even though it was wrecking my life. I was forced to live with it and compelled to care for it like an alien force taking over my mind and body.

But how to describe it? So, so difficult. It went against all the usual rules of illness and if I tried to explain I'd usually end up digging a deeper hole of disbelief.

'How do you feel?'

'Really exhausted.'

'Well, we all feel like that these days. What I do is go for a run.'

'All my limbs and muscles have packed up.'

'Well, that's because you're just sitting around moping. You should find something more stimulating to do, like I do.'

'But my brain doesn't work either.'

'You're obviously depressed. Do try to keep yourself busy, dear.'

'Of course I'm depressed. I can't *do* anything!'

And so it goes on. I just never bothered in the end because I couldn't explain what on earth was happening to me. It was all too scary.

Anyway, I soon realised that my *real* friends could easily see that I was ill – they didn't need an explanation. I dropped the others, who were just using me as a platform to reassure themselves that they weren't failures like me.

And aren't people funny things? Insensitive and selfish could best describe a large group of my former family and so-called friends. Some of them treated me as if I had let them down big time. Firstly, I was inconsiderate enough to get an illness that has no name and no fatality rate and was frowned on by the medical profession.

'Typical of her to get something controversial. Always was a difficult woman.'

If I had been more considerate I should have picked something like cancer – lots of emotional mileage on that one and definitely not an embarrassment.

Secondly, I could no longer be depended on in a crisis, because I was too busy having one of my own. Motionless in my sick bed, I was reminded by visitors how useful I had been to them. I always did this for them and that for them and how on earth did I think they were going to manage now? Surely if I just thought positive and pulled myself together I would be up in a jiffy?

'The thing I miss most about you,' I was told, 'is that no matter how busy you were, you always managed to take us and pick us up from the airport for our holiday and now we can't find anyone to take us even though we're off next week.'

I could see that I'd unwittingly become responsible for other people's problems. Work was the same. I had built on being a problem solver and I knew that I enjoyed and profited from that – but I never expected it to run so deeply in my personal life.

Instead of sympathy, I got anger and guilt trips. To this day I have had no contact with my sister; and my mother refuses to talk about it, maybe because she can't properly name it. What's in a name? A lot, it seems. And although none of them knew what it was, some seemed very keen to give me their opinion about my untimely transformation.

You know, you spend so much effort telling people you aren't depressed, but with this illness you should be! All chronic conditions carry an emotional effect. Of course it is upsetting and frustrating, frightening and demoralising. I felt as if someone had said to me that I might be going to spend the rest of my life a bedridden blob, and I was supposed to turn round and say, 'Oh, goody, at least it's not mental.'

But less of this down talk. Positive thinking does pay! I am left with My Love and a few genuines, whom I would never have found and nurtured in my busy days. I care little about offending a 'past' friend and have no guilt in saying, 'No way, sort it out yourself, I'm far too busy being selfish.'

Take my relationship with my sister. We have never been close and it has always been left to me to keep the relationship going. I can't remember the last time she even bothered to send me a Christmas card, but I always made sure I never forgot any of her family occasions and always called round if I was in the area. Since I've been ill I don't care. She's become less important to me. There's no dislike on my part – it's just the realisation that if she wanted a sister, she would have made it obvious by now. It's far too exhausting trying to please everyone, especially if you expect no return on it.

My bad memory has been a help rather than a hindrance as I can forget the endless months I spent staring at the dead spider on the ceiling – and only small things remind me of the years I've missed. My tape collection in the car is very '93; and all my suits in the wardrobe still have shoulder pads in them, very passé these days. Though by the time I get round to wearing them again, they will be à la mode.

I am far from well, but I am definitely getting better – a phrase I have optimistically used and needed all along. But this time it is true and it is only when you start coming out of this illness that you realise just how poorly you've been.

I look back at major events in my life that are supposed to be the happiest and have to admit they were major only as an ordeal. I tried so hard to join in and 'act normal', but after a few attempts at the social scene I gave up after a disastrous family birthday party.

We had arrived late because I was so ill in the car. I stuck it out in agony for an hour, then borrowed the keys to a friend's house and spent the afternoon in pain, alone and miles from home. When everyone crashed in, drunk and merry, I have never felt so pathetic, clutching my hot water bottle in the corner.

They decided they'd all go clubbing – one of my most

favourite pastimes of old. I was already feeling gutted when a girl turned to me on the way out saying, 'My friend knows this girl who had ME. But she took some Chinese stuff and she's all right now.' Later on in the evening when they'd all gone I cried and cried. But then I was discovered and someone kindly said, 'Look, why not get some anti-depressants, that's what I did.'

That was when I realised it wasn't just my life that ME was destroying. My Love insists he wouldn't want to be anywhere but with me – but I'm sure he'd rather have the Me that he first met, not this brain removed variety.

When I got married last year everyone had a fantastic time, except me. We had planned to keep it small because of my health, my first disappointment, but the day itself was so depressing. I mean, you want to be enjoying yourself, don't you, with all your nearest and dearest, some of whom you haven't seen for ages? But there was no energy there.

I spent all day just concentrating on staying upright. I can't remember any conversations, didn't eat any food and went home to bed at five leaving everyone to have a right good knees-up, including my new husband who crawled in at midnight. I had spent a miserable evening at home, alone, knowing what fun was being had – and how could I begrudge anyone for it? After all I'm the one who is ill, and living with a sick person is no barrel of laughs.

My one saving grace has been My Life, who has loved and cared for me, and I do know how lucky I have been with him. Oh what a sad tale it would have been without his constant devotion. And I mustn't forget Richard and Judy and Supermarket Sweep for getting me through the worst time in the morning!

The only way I have got this far is by treating the whole illness as a job, and my job was to get better. I have tried everything – written to every research hospital, listened to every doctor, tried every alternative health treatment, eaten every type of diet.

I also knew I had to come to terms with my future before I could let go of my past. What was I going to do for money once I had recovered? I had spent years building up my own business and, having lost my income through illness, it wasn't a simple thing to say to myself, 'Well I'm okay now, I can come off benefit and start earning again.' Who was going to employ me? I wasn't going to be able to return to my business again – that safe, unpleasant routine I'd built for myself. I had made the business happen – and now I was going to make my return to health happen.

Someone stopped me in the street the other day – 'I reckon we've all got ME in our house. You know, by the time we get back from work and put the children to bed all we want to do is sleep.'

That's just living life to the full. People with ME can't even start a day – and that's the point people are missing out on.

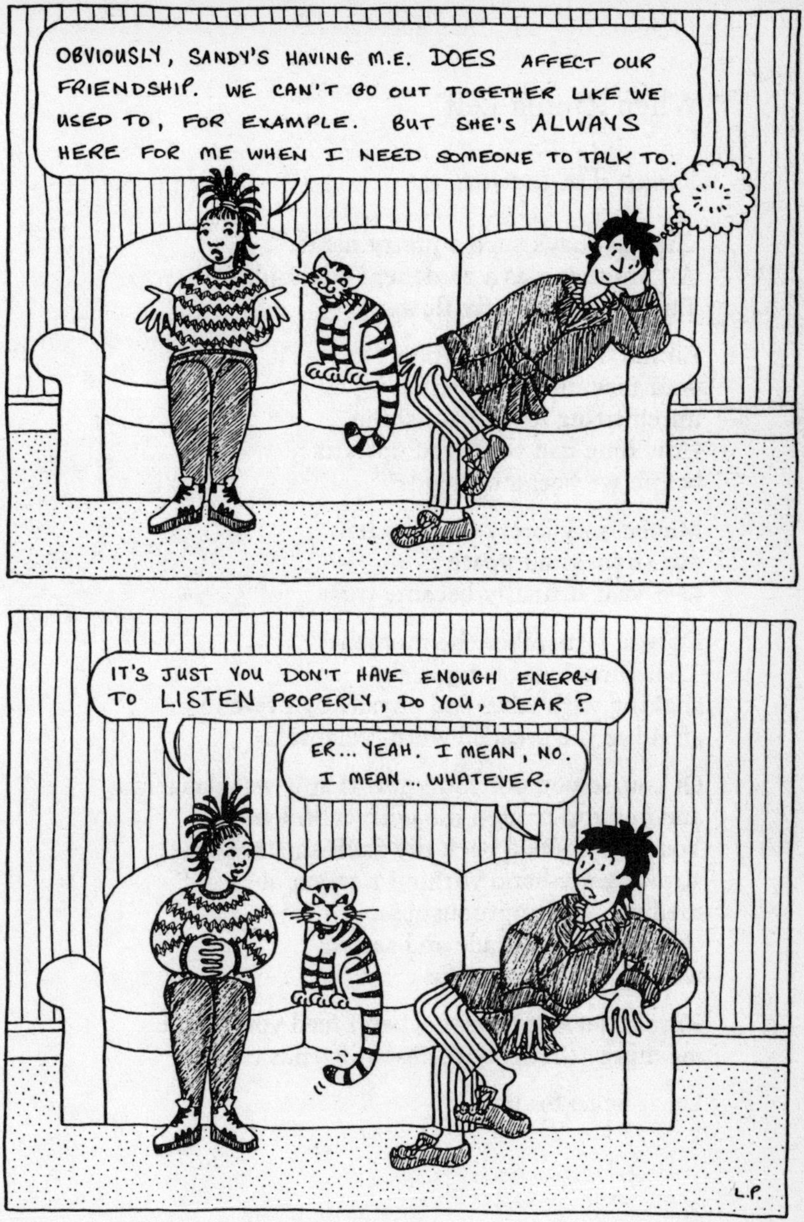
OBVIOUSLY, SANDY'S HAVING M.E. DOES AFFECT OUR FRIENDSHIP. WE CAN'T GO OUT TOGETHER LIKE WE USED TO, FOR EXAMPLE. BUT SHE'S ALWAYS HERE FOR ME WHEN I NEED SOMEONE TO TALK TO.
IT'S JUST YOU DON'T HAVE ENOUGH ENERGY TO LISTEN PROPERLY, DO YOU, DEAR?
ER... YEAH. I MEAN, NO. I MEAN... WHATEVER.
L.P.

When Zinnia Left

Sarah Thompson

'Zinnia, that's such a pretty name.'
'My mother was a gardener,' you said,
'But it's not a pretty flower.'

Zinnia, not like you then,
your face infused with
unremitting love of sunshine.
How long had you lived upstairs
before we became friends?

Maybe only lately I have felt
our shyness dissipate.
Last year it finally became trust.

Do you remember the moment?
That time I was being sick,
shaking with tears and physically overcome,
afraid of the dreaded word, 'relapse'.

Of course you do: you knew that it was dangerous,
and yet you treated me with confidence.
You quietly held back my shell-shocked hair
stroking my hand without a touch of
medical presumptuousness.
Our friendship made and sealed
when pride was at a loss.

Zinnia, I smiled today when I read your name's
meaning: 'thoughts of absent friends'.

Let it be so for us.

To Amanda

Patricia Rock

She enfolds you with her beckoning arms
She lures you away from me
Her hold is stronger than mine
Her grip over you tighter, grasping
Reaching, calling you
Come, come to rest
You need me
Her seductive healing enfolds you
Keeps you alive
Bobbing on the chaos of life.
Yet, I can offer you
Joy, love,
A conscious reality.
When her grasp slackens
You awake
Look about you
On another grey tired day
You're awake!
I've got you back!
For a short while at least.
I know the call will soon come:
Come, come to me
For I will give you
Rest and peace.

Sto Lat Zdrowia

Maria Jastrzębska

Dear Caeia

Thank you for asking me to write something about the Whole Damned Journey, as you put it. I know the kind of piece I would like to write you . . . It would be very wise and the last line would say how I had now completely recovered . . . Is it any wonder I've had trouble getting started ??!

The trouble with chronic illness is that it's chronic. Nothing prepares you for this. I was bewildered when I first became ill. I had never been ill *for so long* before. I want to tell you something about what happened to me and my friends, who were all in some way part of a women's community, a lesbian network.

As lesbians especially we pride ourselves on our independence (financially from men, but in more general terms too). For me strength and physical fitness were of enormous importance. At the time I became ill I was a teacher of self-defence for women and girls. The loss of my physical ability was a terrible blow. Having to learn patience and gentleness has been harder for me than the toughest training I'd ever undergone. Martial artists are awarded belts of varying colours to denote levels of skill and endurance. I would like to see all those with chronic illness similarly decorated – perhaps a different colour for each year.

At the same time as cultivating our toughness to survive in a 'man's world', like most women, many lesbians I know are carers as well, with elderly relatives or with children or both. We are expected to be the givers in society (men the providers). Often we end up being both. Since the lives of lesbians and other 'single' women are often not recognised by our families of origin, even more is expected of us than of our siblings. Our own commitments rarely count.

This is the background against which some of us have become 'mysteriously' ill. When I first became ill with ME, lots of women around me were deciding they'd had enough of self-sacrifice, of over-caring for others and not knowing how to put themselves at the centre of their own lives. Something similar was happening to me. I noticed that the only time I dared put myself first was when I was too ill to do anything else. However, I also needed care *myself*, so it seemed like awful timing if everyone was taking a stand against it. Somehow we ended up in opposite camps. The issues of need and dependence – so complicated for women – came right between us.

Need is a dirty word in the Western world. If you need a ramp in order to get into a building you are seen as a nuisance. If you need a roof over your head, you are treated with suspicion, as some form of low life. In this country even children are not welcomed in many public areas. Those who are ill or frail or vulnerable get shoved into institutions (out of sight) or else are cooped up with one or two equally isolated individuals who are left to cope with little or no support. This is inhuman. It is a daily outrage.

Elsewhere people rely on one another more. At the same time they are faced with such appalling lack of economic and health resources as to make the health service here look like sheer luxury. I am thinking of the inter-dependence among people in countries such as Poland, where I come from, a country only now starting to move towards the First World socially and economically. Whereas in England dependence goes right against the individualistic self-reliance we are supposed to aspire to. Needing help really isn't cricket. This goes deeper than the Thatcher years, though they have contributed hugely. We live in an atomised society, each in our separate units whether as nuclear families, couples or singles. Especially if we live in large cities we rely on our separate gadgets – when we can afford them – and we keep ourselves to ourselves. It's tough to try and go against the grain of that. People are so isolated they burn out, other people's needs then appear a threat, an unbearable burden. But what we think of with embarrassment as our (excessive) needs are in fact basic rights – the same rights that everyone should have.

I was very frightened. My world was shrinking at an alarming rate. My confidence was dwindling. I couldn't do my job. I couldn't keep up with my social life. I was losing all my familiar reference points. I worried that I was becoming boring – I probably was boring. I kept asking why this was happening to me. I grew increasingly self-obsessed, had none of my usual ways of releasing tension or distracting myself from the symptoms which showed no signs of letting up. The relationship I had been in just prior to the onset of the ME had broken up, so I was still getting over that. I knew nothing about services and benefits, such as they are.

Ridley Road, that renowned East London open-air market which I loved, was practically on my doorstep but I was too ill to walk down to it. Friends spouted rhetoric at me about positive thinking; I wondered where my next meal would come from. At that time I didn't know anyone else with ME. There was no end in sight, no shape, nothing to hold on to.

One of the friends I lost was a caring, sensitive woman I had been briefly involved with sexually. Ours was an intense friendship and I always suspected there were some loose ends we had not fully resolved. An excellent listener, she encouraged confidences. She was training to be a healer. In the first months of my illness I leaned on her more than on anyone else. I became more and more dependent till she snapped. The more desperate I felt the more trapped she felt. She said I was making too many demands on her. I felt she didn't know the half of it. I seethed at the thought of her seeing clients on a professional basis while avoiding a close friend who had become so seriously ill. She said I didn't understand the pressures she had in her life. She couldn't keep on top of things for herself, she didn't even have time to get her washing done, let alone deal with my guilt-tripping her. We exchanged angry letters. In the end I suggested we meet to try and sort it out; she refused. Perhaps she thought it was too late for that. She said she wanted to leave behind situations like the one she'd been in with a previous boyfriend. Some time before she had been lovers with a man who had also had a (different) chronic illness. This man had manipulated and guilt-tripped her and in the end become violent and tried to kill her. I was devastated by the comparison – I felt ashamed enough of not recovering – and I gave up.

I envied her her health, but I no longer envied her lifestyle, over-timetabled, overbusy, stressed out. Or that's how it appeared to me. I would look at the lives of other friends too. I'd be horrified at the pressure they seemed to be working and living under – was that how I'd been living? That is one of the true gifts of illness. It did get me to look at the quality of my life. Sometimes we can see more clearly what the so-called healthy life is actually doing to our friends and colleagues and loved ones. More selfishly I wondered how on earth people would ever make room in their busy schedules for me, slow and needy as I felt.

There were similar incidents with other friends. I seemed to have acquired – unbeknown to me – an uncanny ability to remind them of their worst nightmare scenarios of somebody else's illness. More often than not this was parents they had to nurse or take care of when they were too young to be looking after anyone and needed caring for themselves. Occasionally it was a friend or lover, a death, a suicide . . . I had the grim power to summon them all up. I wanted to cry: *but this is me, Maria.*

I wanted to say I understand about this saying no and putting yourself first stuff. It was exactly what I was having to look at in my own life. But there had to be some other way. Switching to the other extreme, distancing ourselves from those 'in need' couldn't be right. Time and time again I saw women give and give and then suddenly decide they'd been too generous. The word on every lesbian's lips seemed to be 'boundary'. I thought if I heard it one more time I'd throw up. Instead of boundaries it seemed as if everyone was putting up barricades and building fortresses around their lives.

My shiatsu practitioner recently asked me how I am around boundaries. I laughed and said, don't you know, Polish people don't have boundaries. As a people we have been invaded, occupied and partitioned. There is literally less space in terms of housing; culturally there is much less 'personal space'. I was brought up to be hospitable and generous to a fault – precious qualities in an age of increasing materialism and greed. But the flip-side is that strain of self-sacrifice. My own family was especially 'close-knit', separated by war and migration from other relatives, we had no choice but to stick together. If someone is ill you make a big fuss of them, cosset and protect them. Friends both Polish and non-Polish can find this 'too much'! To me there is something profoundly kind and refreshingly non-clinical about this approach. However you are also expected to dedicate yourself to caring unreservedly and have no life of your own.

I was shocked I think by my friends' bid for 'freedom' because it went so deeply against the grain of my upbringing (of what I expected to be able to provide for others and what I expected from them when I became ill) but also because there was such an edge to it. There has to be a more balanced, a softer approach. As the West accelerates towards a future which looks increasingly technological, less caring, less human, we surely need to preserve the 'old' values of so-called 'backward' societies without returning to the rigidity and sexism which has restricted women's role to that of sole giver.

Britain is a harsh place. This is not because people here are unkind by nature but because the whole society is being set up to stop us from being kind to one another and to ourselves. It is frightening to become ill (or indeed old) not only because of the physical challenges, but because of the lack of care and respect we face. Our voices have got to be heard if things are to change. This means the voices of the ethnic minorities in this country with our own perspectives on care and the community. It means everyone who is or has been ill *and* everyone looking after somebody ill getting together and having a say.

I used to feel women eyeing me with suspicion, trying to figure out what I might 'need' and quickly throwing up some on the spot barriers. I am writing mostly about friends, because for a long time while I was ill I wasn't involved with anyone sexually. Early on in the illness I did form one new relationship. She was able to see more clearly than me how isolated we both were as a couple. Most lesbian events take place late at night, in smoky, noisy venues. I'd say there is a little more awareness now but not nearly enough of the diversity of women's needs. The cult of (a restricted notion of) youth and the body beautiful doesn't leave much room for difference or vulnerability. The relationship did not last for a variety of reasons; in different ways we were both very vulnerable at the time. This helped us be compassionate towards one another, but at times overwhelmed us. Eventually we were able to retain a friendship, I am glad to say.

Soon after that I nearly lost another friend because I was so scared she'd reject me for being 'too needy' I kept her at arm's length. To my amazement she said she felt rejected by *me*! I couldn't believe it. I'd become so paranoid about people abandoning me, it hadn't occurred to me someone could feel hurt that I was pushing away their help.

I am still cautious about offers of help, though admittedly it is easier to be choosy when you are feeling better. I try to make sure the other person is clear they are doing it for themselves. I don't want a bill or a huge pile of resentment later on. I try to remember they are privileged to be part of my life and to be allowed to give. That's tricky. The stigma of feeling I need 'more' than them – in reality it is not a question of more, but different – is hard to shake off. As soon as it looks like I'm not giving back 'enough', I start to panic. Whatever enough means.

I do not want to give you the impression that all my friendships fell apart when I got ill! But it's often easier to describe the bad times than the good ones. In fact most of my friends have stuck by me, loving me and continuing to hold out hope when I had long lost it. I hope I have done as much for them. They've shown me not only compassion but respect and keep on reminding me that there is more to me than my illness. They have been honest about how my illness affects them. Many, many friends have given me practical help when they could, from cooking (even enough to freeze for later!) and endless shopping to typing poems, driving the cat to the vet, helping me move house, more driving, painting and decorating. New friendships have formed, old ones deepened. Some women have had experiences of illness of their own and are perhaps less horrified by the thought of vulnerability. By some act of grace we've managed to show each other our love even when we have not had the resources to do anything at all for one another. We have found ways to say: I am still here. We have refused to cut off or give up on each other.

I wish I could tell you that later on when I was feeling stronger and met others 'worse off', iller than myself, I was wise to all this. Well, I was aware of the process. But I've got the same over-caring habits as the next girl. How could I be feeling better if they were still ill . . . It wasn't their demands (mostly they'd be too terrified to make any), it was the *thought* of them which overwhelmed me. Instantly I became the only one in the world with the job of personally saving them. I'd forget they had friendship to offer me and that I could expect something back from them. I'd catch myself being as patronising as people had been towards me: how could I ask anything of them when they were *so ill*?! I *OUGHT* to be giving to them . . . of course that way of thinking took the pleasure right out of giving. Thankfully, they've had the courage to challenge me and not let me run away.

In the first couple of years of my illness I had emphatically stated that I 'intended' to recover – it is there in the author's notes of every publication I was involved with. After some years had gone by the whole notion of recovery seemed like a farce. Feeling better, I started saying the 'r' word again. Another relapse came and I gave up again. So it went on. Recently I've had glimmers of what recovery might look like. I can only tell you it is a tiny spark and I can't see it the whole time, but for a very long time it was not there at all.

Everyone likes a happy ending – I'm no exception. Right now it is just over eight years since I became ill, though in fact I'd had periods of lesser illness which I believe led up to this. I believe the worst is behind me, not least because I now know the ropes. I will never be as isolated again. I know I am one of countless people living with an illness or disability and it is another of the gifts of this illness to feel connected to them in some way. I still have much to learn. But other ill and disabled people will never be 'Them' to me as they once were and for that I am grateful. I feel that I occupy a place between health and sickness. At times I am among the healthy and the ME is fairly invisible. I usually look well, so I 'pass' as such. It is a strange position. I no longer try every latest miracle cure. Perhaps it's the despair at work. But I don't want to focus on the illness any more than I have to. My energy goes on interests which take my mind off it. My writing has always been a way through. It's a stroke of luck for me that writing is less physically demanding than other passions in my life, though many times I have simply been too ill to write.

I am now in one of the best relationships I have ever had. Not only do I have the everyday support of an incredibly loving and non-judgemental partner, but I have the joy of loving her and feeling how much I have to give again, to her, to her daughter, to those around me. The challenge facing us – probably like any couple – is not to take one another for granted. Of course it is easier to ask D for help and there is a danger of us getting isolated with the illness (as indeed with any problem). I have therapy and am involved with co-counselling. I am doing everything I can to create an environment in which my spirit thrives and one in which illness squirms and fades. Getting the right balance between rest (so crucial for ME'rs) and excitement, without which life becomes unbearable, is a constant puzzle. I take risks and push at my limits. I cower and dread any change to my routine. I get scared leaving the house, but I've been abroad. I still overdo it. I still find it excruciating to ask for help, despite all this wonderful practice. That terrible sense of shame still washes over me. As if I just wasn't trying hard enough. I have never met a single soul who had ME and didn't try to get better with all their heart. Where does this cruel notion come from of us wanting to be ill? It is so clearly another version of that 'she asked for it', blame the victim, mentality – yet I still struggle with it.

One of the hardest things I find is continuing to look after myself when I am in a 'better' phase. In a sense, paradoxically, this is when I am most at risk. This is the time when I find it difficult to say no to anything. After all, I'm all right now, I *should* be able to cope. That's exactly when I need to carry on giving myself treats and rests and making sure I am following my heart rather than slotting in to fit anyone else's expectations or social pressures. But there is this belief system which says you don't deserve any care unless you are really suffering. It's what I call the 'I'm fine/I don't need anything (anyone)/Good Work-Horse Syndrome'. Spotting it and actively challenging it is essential preventative medicine.

I practise this medicine any chance I get. My life has changed enormously since I first got ill. I'm not sure I've found a cure, but I am certainly healing inside. I no longer live in a small inner city flat with no garden. I live in a house in Brighton, so as to be closer to the sea and the countryside. There are now children and cats in my life. A patio full of plants, gulls squawking overhead. Some of this is down to pure luck, some of it is privilege and some perseverance on my part. And as all the self-help books tell you, the kinder I am to myself the more I have to give others and the more of a pleasure it is. Does this sound too rosy? Well, it isn't all sweetness and light, I can assure you. But you and everyone else involved with this book are there. All of us. We are not alone, not only in struggling for our health, but in wishing for, demanding, praying for or campaigning for a world in which we can truly be healed, in which no one is deemed not cost-effective or relegated to the human scrap heap, in which the frailest amongst us is cherished and treated with complete respect.

Sto lat zdrowia (a hundred years of health),
love, Maria.

Loving Woman

Aspen

You come to me
loving woman
with kindness and promise
filling with warmth
my open spaces
making me carefree
with dizzy smiles.

You know I want
this freedom I feel
you know I want
my ill body to soar
in comfort and safety
to race with the clouds
and sing with the wind.

We float down to rest
your warm arms chase
the ghosts of doubts,
words cannot express
this soul-love-song
which rushes like torrents
through all my veins.

We are made of
courage and tenderness
as I touch your
dark, wild hair
my body discovers
such soft warmth
as we spin dancing
through the night.

Part Three

Healing Ourselves

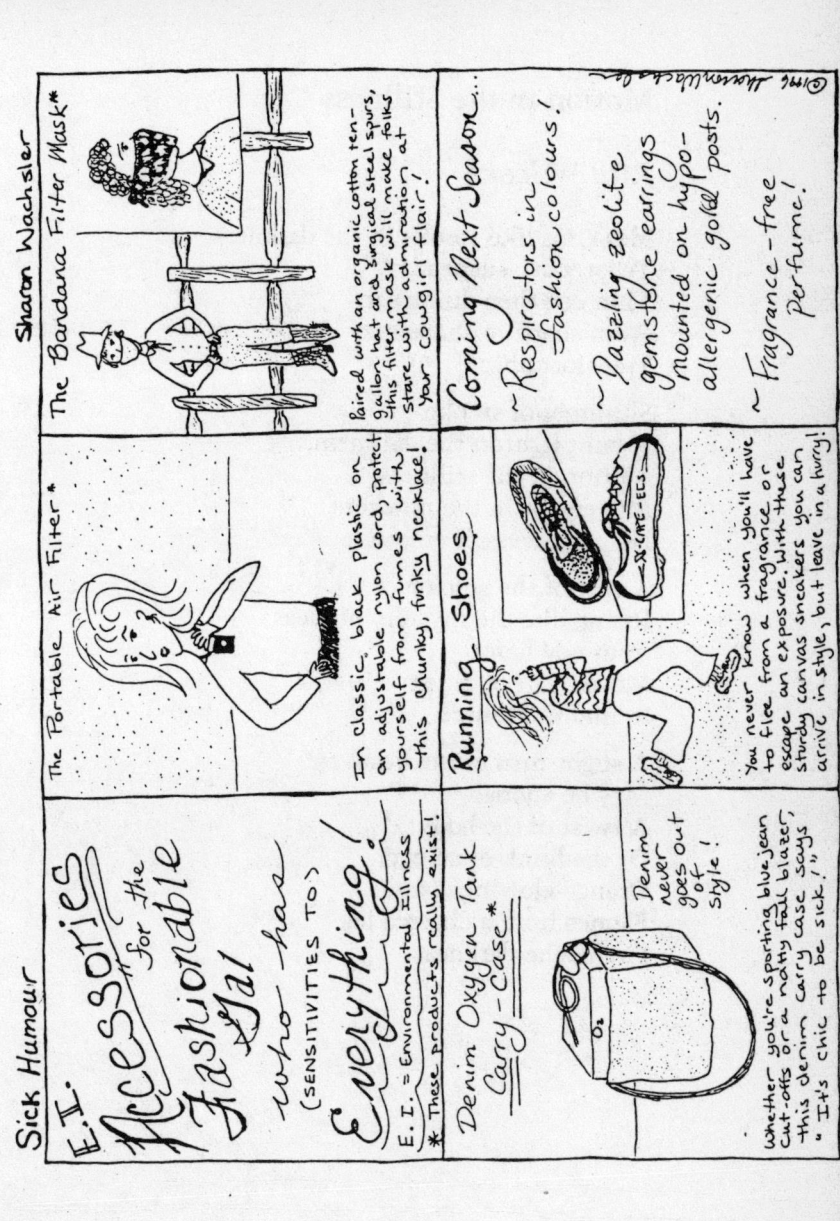

Sick Humour

Sharon Wachsler

E.I.
Accessories
for the
Fashionable
Gal
who has
(SENSITIVITIES TO)
Everything!

E.I. = Environmental Illness
* These products really exist!

The Portable Air Filter *

In classic, black plastic on an adjustable nylon cord, protect yourself from fumes with this chunky, funky necklace!

The Bandana Filter Mask*

Paired with an organic cotton ten-gallon hat and surgical steel spurs, this filter mask will make folks stare with admiration at your cowgirl flair!

Denim Oxygen Tank Carry-Case *

Denim never goes out of style!

Whether you're sporting blue jean cut-offs or a natty full blazer, this denim carry case says "It's chic to be sick."!

Running Shoes

SX-LIME-EES

You never know when you'll have to flee from a fragrance or escape an exposure. With these sturdy canvas sneakers you can arrive in style, but leave in a hurry!

Coming Next Season...

~ Respirators in fashion colours!

~ Dazzling zeolite gemstone earrings mounted on hypo-allergenic gold posts.

~ Fragrance-free perfume!

© 1996 Sharon Wachsler

Motion in the Stillness

Rita Wilcock

Ideas rise like smoke in the darkness.
Twist, curl, suspend,
Thin out then disappear.
From shape to shapeless,
Transforming.

Shimmer of smoke
A faint light in the darkness.
Motion in the stillness,
Movement in the nowhere,
No awareness of emotion.

Aware of the smoke
Rising like the mystery of ideas
from nowhere.
Move, wait or listen
to find the source.

A slight turn of the head
May be enough
A twist of the body
Or the blink of an eye.
Orange-glowing coals,
Flames from a charred log
Fire in the darkness.

Just a Teensy Weensy Bit Defiant

Andrea Goodman

My quest for healing has taken me on a wonderful journey to myself. Let's face it, there is nothing like chronic illness to break down our barriers and expose our inner being in all its vulnerability, and this certainly happened to me. My biggest problem was coming to terms with the fact that I was no longer the outgoing, dynamic bundle of energy that revelled in life; suddenly I was this totally alien being, completely sapped of energy and full of aches, pains and angst. I was a blob mostly confined to my bed, unable to function physically or mentally and convinced that I was going mad.

The isolating aspect of this condition gave me plenty of time to think and naturally my thoughts were centred around what I needed to do in order to recover my health. My GP offered me kindness and 'pep talks' but little else. Eventually, after weeks of scrutinising my sorry situation it dawned on me that this total disintegration of my life was a perfect mirror of my inner self. Not only was I physically ill, but my whole being ached, and I realised that to truly recover my full health I had to tackle it on every level – physically, mentally/emotionally and spiritually. Once I had this realisation my outlook was transformed. I was not prepared to take on the role of victim despite the odds against me. Some four months later was to be my first success. I was well enough to start the recovery plan I had devised.

My first priority was to get some help for my somewhat feeble body. I heard about the Centre for Complementary Medicine in Southampton and duly booked myself an appointment. They use vega testing as a means to find imbalances in the body. Needless to say I had lots of those –

nutritional deficiencies, candida, kidney imbalance, and so many allergies that the diet sheet given to me excluded so many foods that my weight plummeted. Also my blood was tested for magnesium levels that turned out to be too low to be helped by orally administered magnesium, and so I had injections which gave me a real boost physically. Muscle twitching stopped and I had a marked increase in my energy levels. After a few weeks of treatment the candida had gone and all the allergies except one had disappeared. The treatment consisted of herbal tablets for the candida, mega doses of various vitamins, fish oils, Ginkgo biloba, folic acid – the list is endless and so were the tablets I swallowed. The treatment did improve my health but once I stopped having treatment due to financial considerations my health deteriorated again, though not to the point where I was again bedridden. Needless to say the treatment is not available on the NHS. However, my energy levels were much improved so I could also concentrate on other areas of my life.

My greatest need at that point was to find some way of nourishing myself spiritually. Traditional religious institutions have never appealed to me so I looked further afield. At this time I discovered the North American Indian tradition and the Goddess traditions and attended occasional workshops to learn about their beliefs. I soon discovered that to gain anything at all I had to engage myself wholeheartedly in quiet meditation, to enter into the silence and allow the answers to come to me. These precious times exhausted me but I received so much from them in terms of self-awareness and my connection with all things that the experiences live in me still – it isn't something that gets put back in a box.

I started occasionally writing poems and prayers. The awakening spiritual qualities within me were inspired by the wonderful mythology of yesteryear. I was particularly struck by the Isis legend, she who symbolises the feminine creative power, who is courageous, who falls deep into the abyss of despair and desolation, confronts her 'demons' both within and without and emerges triumphant – whole and balanced. How I wanted that for me.

Just a Teensy Weensy Bit Defiant 127

Isis

January 1994

May her presence be known to me
May her presence quieten me
May her presence nurture me
May her presence sustain me
May her presence lift the rainbow veil between the two worlds
May her presence bring me strength;
the strength to find the woman I can be
May her presence bring me courage;
the courage to be that woman
May her presence fill me with love;
love enough to be me

And so my road to recovery lay before me, a friend
reminding me 'little steps, tiny little steps' when frustration
at my lack of progress set in, as days turned to weeks and
months with no signs of improvement. However, little by
little I did grow stronger, inwardly at first until suddenly I
realised a new level of well-being had been attained. Now it
was the end of 1995 – four years of struggle were behind me.

After a minor operation in January 1996 my physical
health deteriorated to such an extent that most of the day
was spent resting and my digestive system broke down –
general anaesthetic is not kind to ME sufferers. At this point
I hit an all-time low mentally, believing that all my hard
work had amounted to nothing. Life was playing a cruel joke
on me and I wanted to die. There was just no way that I
could possibly go through the last few years again, and so I
entered the silence and asked the powers above to release
me from this world. Obviously they didn't indulge me in my
wish to go home as it were, but that night I had a very
powerful dream that in some way gave me the strength to
get off my self-pitying butt and do something about it. I can't
describe how angry I was that this should happen to me
again! (I wrote the dream in the form of a poem.)

Death

February 1996

Death comes to me like a lover, young and beautiful
Dancing around me, teasing, flaunting herself
The waiting is agonising and I try to grab her, grasping at
   death
She twists out of my hands running towards the wind, a
   whirling dervish
in the distance, laughing hollow laughter that turns to
   howling and shrieking

She is no longer the young lover, time peels away the
   layers
and I am confronted by the hidden face of the Goddess
It is not possible to gaze upon the face of this Goddess
Her eyes are recesses of a raging inferno
Her presence is terrible, blood turns to stone
Even time stands still in fear of the monster I have
   unleashed

She has cheated me again, Death has cheated me again
Her wailing summons up the ghosts of all my lives, the
   ghosts of all my misdemeanours
Am I not but the sum total of them
Does not the law of Karma dictate that and doesn't my
   physical being live it
Is death not laughing at me
We must die to live and in facing death
I must find a reason to live – I'm still looking

Through all this I have had the support of a very special and
dear friend who sat with me through the dark times,
encouraged me, supported me and laughed with me when
there was nothing else we could do. She found an article
about Chinese herbal medicine and its success with ME. My
first appointment was towards the end of February, and after
a couple of weeks my health improved dramatically. Now it
is July 1996 I am still taking the herbs and physically I feel

so good. Although I'm still not completely recovered I am able to participate in all sorts of activities and take great pleasure in filling my days with furniture-decorating, voluntary work, anything that is non-stressful and creative! My greatest joy in this vein is being able to play the guitar again. Also for the first time in years I am looking at the future and feeling excited about the possibilities, and if I am honest, a little scared too. I know my days of chronic illness are in the past and I feel free. I'm finding a new way of being, a way that supports and nurtures me, and here I am stout-hearted, strong-willed and just a teensy weensy bit defiant.

The Things That Have Helped Turn ME Around

Shelley Pielou

There must be any number of publications giving the basic information about ME – that it may be caused by a virus (always a trigger word to make doctors glaze over with a sudden attack of vagueness and 'maybes'); that rest is the prime remedy, followed by a brief rest, after which be a devil and just for variety try some more rest. No alcohol, forget smoking and sex can be tricky. Ho, ho, ho. Not feeling a touch *depressed*, are you? Better not let any passing psychiatrist pick up on *that* or you'll be filed under P for psychiatric case rather than M for myalgic before you can say 'applying for DLA is like the search for the Holy Grail – long, arduous but ultimately rewarding'.

This is about the other bits of arcane ME person's information that it's taken me years to discover. All revealed in the hope you may not have to struggle on quite as long as I did (19 years) before you can start to describe yourself as *'recovering from ME'*. I seem to have passed effortlessly from being 'tragically young to be chronically ill, blighted in her prime' etc., to being pre-menopausal, never having *had* a prime. But I'm not bitter. Not much – as in, is the Pope a Catholic?

These are the things that have helped turn me around:

1. I got rid of any abusive relationships or letting people exhaust me or put me down. I read books on co-dependency (basically defined as taking too much care of others and too little of yourself), especially *Codependent No More*[1] and *The Language of Letting Go*[2], both by Melody Beattie. I faced some losses but the reality was that a good, nurturing, mutually respectful relationship with any of these people was lost long before. It was just a question of facing it and

cutting out the dead wood from my life. Yes, it did include leaving my partner; no, I have not got into another relationship; yes, the excruciating pain did pass and no, I don't regret it.

2. I changed my value system. I really kicked and screamed inwardly against this one (see point 3). I had been an actress and single-minded to the point of ruthlessness when it came to my career. But I finally got to the point that hanging on to valuing myself (or not doing so) based on what I could achieve today, as opposed to valuing myself for being a unique human being and irreplaceable was causing me a lot of grief for no gain. It means I do my best to value everyone else equally, on the basis of *their* uniqueness and humanity, rather than mentally placing everyone on a scale somewhere above or below me. I still get the occasional attack of this, but I've now learned to stop the thought in its tracks and try to see what it is that has turned me back into a competitor, not a co-operator. It's usually fear-based and comes from old useless messages from the part of my life that set me up for ME. So I try to let it go and replace it with accepting myself and other people as just fine the way I am and they are.

3. I discharge hostility. I think it's absolutely essential. Having been initiated into the dreary requirements of patriarchy ('I don't expect anger from you, Shelley' was a family classic), I have plenty to discharge and unlearn. But letting it out by screaming unsettles me and punching a pillow can be really exhausting and painful. So I *visualise* screaming, kicking and generally beating the crap out of either my pillow or the offending person. Then I soothe myself down by visualising something peaceful like being massaged, and so get free of emotions that do take a lot of energy to suppress without spilling too much energy getting them out. Stream-of-consciousness writing and drawing about what's going on (strictly for my own consumption) really help too, and again I try and create a feeling of peacefulness at the end by drawing myself as a serene figure

nurturing the suffering part of me or whatever feels right.

4. I use Jin Shin Jyutsu, a system of self-help acupressure that I learned from a practitioner, Roselyn Journeaux. She is inspiring, having recovered from ME herself and being now outstandingly fit and working ten hours a day. She is also sensitive and aware of the responsibility involved in treating very ill people. (Something that cannot be said for all the alternative practitioners I've tried. I've found this to be an important element: that anyone I consult as well as being thoroughly trained, with an approach that does work with ME, is also aware of my physical and emotional vulnerability in going to them, and always obeys the first principle of 'do no harm'.) Roselyn has worked steadily with me for several years, gradually building up the self-help treatment I give myself, with a boost from being treated by her once a month. Acupressure is a bit like acupuncture without the needles and does not require pressure but simply resting fingers on the appropriate pressure points. By lying down with my arms propped on pillows to do Jin Shin, my arm muscles don't get sore.

5. I use Chinese food herbs for maximum nutritional value and safety. The ones I use are produced in California, subject to US food and drug safety laws which are more stringent than those in Britain. Maybe I'm having an attack of Californian schmalz but I love these Sunrider herbs, or rather I love the changes they are bringing about in me. I resisted taking herbs for a long time, glad of the benefits from the Jin Shin and not wanting to rock the metabolic boat. I chose the formula that helps to regenerate the adrenals, reproductive glands, liver, pancreas, kidneys and the nervous system. Recently, I have introduced Fortune Delight tea as well, a de-toxifier which boosted my energy (but gently – no speedy over-stimulation); and also Quinary herbs, so named because they support the five major systems of the body.

I am increasingly relying on these herbs[3] and have reduced the large doses of vitamins that I previously relied on in order to function at all. The herbs are expensive at first sight, but over the long haul they are not much more costly than paying prescription charges each month. And in my case, they have done my ME far more good than anything I ever obtained on prescription.

6. I stroke my cat. The therapeutic benefits of stroking a pet are well known, and my cat is a loyal and trusty supporter in living with ME. Being ill is often isolating and there is a great comfort in giving and receiving affection from someone who is always there, always uncritically pleased to see you. At one point my cat was not uncritically pleased to see me. I realised that chronic illness had dampened my spirits and that I was omitting to play with him. I dosed him with some Bach Flower remedies to ease his feeling of rejection: I chose the ones for being aloof and depression of unknown origin. I bought him some cat toys and we both cheered up a lot.

I resisted getting a pet for a long time, and went into all the pros and cons before I did. Possible arguments against include the cost of veterinary treatment and the cost of food. I live in London so there are branches of the RSPCA, Blue Cross and other animal charities in my area. The RSPCA branch nearby treats animals for free and you donate what you can afford. Whiskers was originally a stray, so a charity, Animal Aid, neutered him free of charge; or I could have got a voucher to cover the cost of neutering from the Cats' Protection League. When a friend had to go into hospital, the Cinnamon Trust, a wonderful charity operating across the country, provided a volunteer to look after her pet while she was an in-patient. As for the cost of food – cats don't eat that much and mine often enjoys leftovers. The increase of joy he brings into my life more than outweighs the cost. Watching Whiskers, whose figure definitely does not equip him for the corps de ballet, more like the corpulent ballet, spiral, leap and pirouette as he chases passing flies, autumn leaves and contemptuous pigeons can make me laugh out loud and lightens my day at home.

7. I finally faced the reality that I should stop eating things that disagree with me. It's just not worth the momentary pleasure for the hours of misery that can follow.

This is a highly individual matter, but for me it meant cutting out all dairy products, yeast, sugar, chocolate, tea and coffee and red meat, as all seemed to result in a general worsening of symptoms, including diarrhoea and low blood sugar. I had been interpreting all my irritable bowel-type symptoms as caused solely by food, and so was cutting out everything that seemed to cause problems until last year I wound up in hospital a stone underweight. The nurses assumed I was anorexic and bullied me into introducing more foods into my diet, and that was how I discovered that living solely on fish and millet or buckwheat, vegetable casserole, oatcakes and grapefruit was neither necessary nor a good idea.

So now I steer a middle path and eat a much more varied and delicious diet, while staying away from what are for me the real hooligan foods that just vandalise my digestion otherwise. Linusit organically grown cracked linseeds soaked in water then eaten with yoghurt has helped the symptoms of IBS. An anti-candida diet does help me, along with a supplement of BioCare's Mycopryl.

8. I have consulted a lot of healers, with results ranging from mild temporary improvement and feeling encouraged to being in a lather of fury at some misinformed, ineptly applied New Age claptrap. I find it a lot more helpful if healers perform laying-on of hands and listen, rather than trying – in however well-intentioned a way – to explain some spiritual 'cause' for my illness.

9. I use transcendental meditation (TM). It is one of the few verified treatments for ME. An 'Action for ME' leaflet on the use of relaxation and meditation for people with ME described TM as being a powerful relaxant of both body and mind, with concomitant benefits. I had great difficulty with any form of relaxation until I learned TM – as soon as I tried to listen to a relaxation tape or to think 'my arms are heavy'

my heart would start to pound and I would feel myself start to speed up inwardly. TM broke this pattern. I find it can revive me with its combination of deep mental and physical relaxation so that the last few hours of the afternoon are enjoyable, not an exhausted fog. Unfortunately learning TM is expensive and certainly my local centre stopped offering concessions for the unwaged some time ago. But I was able to pay in instalments starting from when I learned, so being on a tight budget should hopefully not prevent any interested person from taking up TM.

10. Last but not least – I am developing my spiritual side. It helped a lot when someone said to me, 'Why don't you choose your own concept of God?' That cleared a lot of unwanted received ideas out of the way and set me free to find what's right for me. I hope this process will continue for the rest of my life. I am prayed for, too, albeit by women whose religion I do not adhere to. It feels really supportive to know it happens.

Other things which helped me, but which there's not time or space to go into, include:
* Aromatherapy massage.
* Homeopathy (from a practitioner, not self-prescribing).
* Co-counselling – a system of counselling by lay people whereby you take a 'Fundamentals' course, usually one evening a week for two months, learning to listen and give feedback, and can then start to share co-counselling sessions with a fellow co-counsellor, taking it in turns to be the person being counselled. I could not have coped with this when I was bed-bound or feeling too vulnerable to give support to someone else, but otherwise it can be an excellent, low-cost way of obtaining counselling and having an opportunity to give something back. I found it a great boost to my self-esteem to realise I had something to give instead of only needing help.
* I eat organically grown vegetables (if you get what's in season, it's less expensive).

* I eat the vegetables raw on the occasions when I am constipated and have them cooked if I'm the other way round.
* I got a water filter: unfiltered tap water can contain a lot of nasties like nitrates and heavy metals.
* Although I love staying up late, I go to bed by 10 pm. The best quality sleep is apparently obtained between 10 pm and 1.00 am. I take ages to get ready for bed so it means starting to get ready at 9.00 pm, but when I manage to do it (not that often, I have to admit), the results more than outweigh the irritants.
* I don't have a TV in the bedroom (having one in there made me much more ill).
* I try not to have electric cables running across the wall at the head of my bed. Since they are there where I live at present and moving the bed is not practicable, I turn them off while I sleep.
* I don't use an electric blanket. (These last three items I assume all relate to problems caused by electro-magnetism. I don't understand *why* making these changes has helped me, I only know that it has made me feel better.)
* I have a nightlight candle in an aromatherapy oil burner with a few drops of lavender oil in it burning while I sleep – breathing in the relaxing scent can improve the quality of sleep and dreaming. And the light is comforting as I take a long time to fall asleep and tend to wake up during the night. I find that lavender cheers me up if I am depressed (especially if mixed with a few drops of geranium) and, paradoxically, calms me down if I am high. But be warned that reactions to essential oils vary and are dose related – I never take them internally and I started off with three drops in the oil burner building up to a maximum of six drops after I had checked out my reaction to lavender.
* I have lots of pillows to sit propped up on while I'm in bed – they are very cheap at Woolworth's and Argos and give me a small sense of luxury.
* I remind myself that living with chronic illness throws me back on resources most people never discover if they possess

or not. I try not to put myself down for the weepy despairing times, but instead to put my arms around myself in a big hug and say 'I'm precious and worthwhile and courageous' – because I am. And if you are surviving living with the rigours of ME, then so too are you.

Notes
1. Beattie, Melody, *Codependent No More*, Hazelden (Educational Materials), 1989.
2. Beattie, Melody, *The Language of Letting Go*, Hazelden, 1990. Also on cassette at £9.99, 1994.
3. Finnegan J, and Gray, Daphne, *Recovery from Addiction*, see chapter on 'Nutritional Therapies',' Celestial Arts, Berkeley, California, USA. Available from Compendium Bookshop, Camden, North London (tel. 0171 485 8944).

All other resources mentioned here are listed in Part Three of the Resources List.

The Visit

Kay Bastin

I'm sitting in front of a greying middle-aged man who reeks of aftershave and money. He is as patronising as hell. What am I, a self-respecting feminist, doing here? I'm under the care of the National Health Service. I'm hoping this 'expert' will give me some help and advice about my ME. But he has already decided what is wrong with me before I set foot in the room.

'Your doctor says that you're weepy. So you're depressed, then.'

I am well-trained. I am a union steward. I negotiate with people like this. I answer calmly: .

'No, I'm not "depressed". I was upset when she told me I had ME, and I'm pissed off with being ill.'

. . . Suddenly there's this Amazon leaping around wielding an axe . . .

'YOU STUPID BASTARD!! YOU'D BE UPSET IF YOUR LIFE HAD JUST BEEN TURNED UPSIDE-DOWN!!'

. . . The axe swings. Blood drips on to his nice white coat.

He is explaining in a bored voice:

'. . . the main factors are emotional and psychological . . .'

I stare at him:

'Are you saying that this is all in my head?'

It is clear he doesn't believe in ME, at all.

She's doing a war-dance on his scalp . . .

'OK BUSTER, LET'S HAVE A LOOK AT WHAT'S IN YOUR HEAD, SHALL WE??'

He tries another tack:

'Have you always been this heavy?'

I smile at him as if he's just paid me a huge compliment,

'Yes, I was a chubby child.'

'HEAVY!! I'LL GIVE YOU HEAVY . . .'
. . . She drops a large concrete block on him. He collapses like a concertina.

He examines me. His fingers feel my generous belly with distaste. He retreats to my feet to test my reflexes.

'OFF WITH THOSE PATRIARCHAL PHALANGES!!'
. . . His heavy gold initialled signet ring rolls on to the floor.

He pronounces judgment:
'You are depressed.'
I grit my teeth.
'I've already said I disagree. No doubt that'll go in my notes as "denies depression".'
He's not listening:
'. . . and I think you should take anti-depressants. We'll discuss your management next time.'

She cleaves his desk in two with one blow . . .
'PAY ATTENTION, PAL!! SHE SAID "NO!!"
. . . and she whips up a tornado that hurls him around the room in a clutter of papers and instruments.
We leave him slumped in a corner whimpering:
'I will not patronise women . . . I will not patronise women . . . I will not patronise women . . .'

Inscribed on his desk is a reminder:

WE'LL BE BACK . . .

We walk arm in arm down the corridor. Heads turn, a hush falls . . . Well, let's face it, it's not often you see a six-foot axe-toting Amazon in a hospital, now is it?

I wrote 'The Visit' after a visit to the consultant that left me feeling utterly frustrated and powerless. It was good 'therapy' and it was great fun! I now firmly believe in taking an Amazon to every medical appointment. Actually the possibilities are endless: the bank, the mortgage, the DSS and every benefits agency doctor should definitely be Amazoned!

When I first became ill my GP at the time, who believed in early diagnosis for ME, sent me to a consultant who, it became apparent, did not believe in ME! He started with 'Depression', moved on to 'Menopause', briefly acknowledged the possibility of a 'Post-viral state' when my results came back, returned to 'Depression' and added 'Lupus', a serious disease, without any counselling or advice. I 'sacked' him at this point, having finally accumulated enough energy to get angry.

The next consultant believed in ME, and was very sympathetic, but sent his patients to physio for 'aerobic exercises'. So there I was, a physio myself, waddling slowly into the department where I used to work, knowing full well that they were watching my 'gait', how I sat down, how I got up, and feeling as apprehensive as any patient. Around me I could hear people being encouraged to do more, work harder. The thought crossed my mind, terrifyingly: 'And what are they going to make me do?' (Did I really do that once? Make people do things like that?)

I gave the physio my 'history' and listened meekly as she described the exercises she wanted me to do, building up to 15 minutes a day (??!!) and how next time I would go on the exercise bike – no resistance on it (I should think not!) – to have my oxygen intake measured. I was exhausted just thinking about it . . . And for what reason? Because *someone* has decided that aerobic exercise is good for ME, and *someone* is doing a study to prove it. Not on me, they're not. This physio is breaking ranks. I'll get my aerobic exercise going upstairs, opening the curtains, or just putting my shoes on . . . And what I need is a good community physio and occupational therapist to sit down and discuss with me ways of managing how I am, and how to avoid stiffening up. It's called real life.

HEY LADIES! Want to DROP those unsightly pounds?

TRY THE CFIDS* DIET©!

* Chronic Fatigue Immune Dysfunction Syndrome

That's right! You've __failed__ with other weight-loss techniques: starving yourself, exercising fanatically, bingeing on grapefruit... NOW there's a _natural_ way to achieve the wasting required for the fashionable "Waif" look!

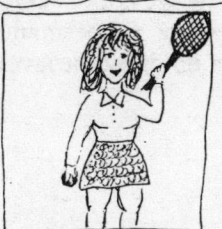

Before...

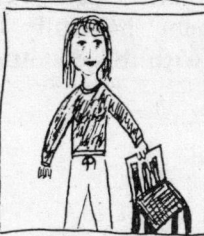

After!

© Sharon Wachsler 1996

You'll Get:
~ Nausea...
~ Diarrhoea...
~ Appetite loss...
~ Fevers...
~ and much more!

"I felt like I was dying, but my friends and family couldn't get over how __great__ I looked!"

NO DIFFICULT EXERCISES!!

ACT NOW and for NO EXTRA CHARGE you can get multiple chemical sensitivities and food allergies!! No more impromptu trips to the store! Kiss these bulky, calorie-laden foods good-bye: chocolate, dairy, soy, wheat, __and up to 100 additional foods!__

"you'll never look at food the same way again!"

The Labyrinth

Linda Newton

My journey through the labyrinth of healers/therapists and treatments continually returned me to the mind/body connection. Every cell of my body held an innate intelligence for healing; if I could tap into this force I could initiate positive changes for my good health. Ultimately, it has to be Nature that heals; I needed to create a fertile environment for this to occur.

Along with my herbalist, Mr W, I knew we could achieve sustained improvement, hopefully leading to permanent recovery, by dealing with this condition on different levels:

- the physical
- the emotional
- the psychological
- the intellectual
- the spiritual

Here are the techniques, measures and therapies I employed to encourage my mind, body and spirit back to good health.

Diet

Under the advice and guidance of Mr W I looked very closely at my diet; he emphasised, very strongly, the health benefits of sticking to a balanced diet. *We are what we eat.* Look at plants that have been properly fed and nurtured; they radiate with energy and health. We are no different. I did not make radical changes overnight, as that would have upset my system; however, over a period of months:

I cut out of my diet, completely red meat; coffee; white bread; fizzy, canned drinks; fried, fatty foods. *I substantially reduced my intake of:* sweets; cakes; pastries; processed foods; margarine; dairy products; strong tea. *I increased my intake of:* fresh fruit; fresh vegetables; salad stuffs; wholemeal bread; chicken; fresh fish; pulses; pasta; brown rice; herbal teas.

Once a healthier diet had been established I felt more energised, and my body felt stronger inside.

Massage/Hugging

I had a weekly massage, given to me by a qualified therapist. It was a very gentle massage, given that my muscles ached, but it did help me relax. I had to re-educate myself to ask people for a hug; if I was unable to get a hug from a person I settled for my old 'Teddy' nightdress case.

Laughter

Once I began to feel more centred and in control of my own recovery, I discovered that I still had the ability to laugh. My eyes were still very sensitive, so rather than watch the television I listened to old cassette tapes: *The Navy Lark*, *Jimmy Clitheroe*, and *Round the Horne*. Laughter had a direct effect on my immune system, so I continued to exercise my chuckle muscle with a daily dose of comedy.

Painting

I am a lousy artist, but I bought some pots of poster paints, brushes, and huge sheets of paper, and I painted and I painted. Initially, the pictures were very bizarre, and mainly black and red, but as I continued to paint I began using soothing blues and greens. I am convinced that tapping into this creative side of my personality was very cathartic for me.

Exercise

About six months after my consultation with Mr W I felt strong enough to attempt a little exercise; my ability varied from day to day, so I adjusted my programme accordingly. The exercises were always very gentle, rather like yoga –

gentle stretching and bending. If I had a 'down' day, I did not include exercises in my activities.

Relaxation

During my illness I had spent significant periods of time in bed, supposedly 'resting'. However, because of the frustration and complexity of my symptoms, along with the constant battle to get my condition identified, I had been unable to achieve any true level of relaxation. Once I set about this in a more positive way (spurred on by the herbal medication) I discovered that I responded most effectively to Baroque music, which I listened to daily for 20 minutes or so.

I avoided playing the heart-wrenching stuff that I had listened to previously; it was too emotive, personally, to relax to. Later on I acquired some 'rainforest' music, complete with all the sound effects; it was quite amazing. Overall, this helped me to acquire and maintain a sense of 'inner calm'.

Decoration and Atmosphere

I stuck pictures/photos of ordinary, everyday folk, smiling, laughing, having fun, all over the flat. Smiles, like yawns, are highly contagious. I also managed to acquire several plants that needed little or no attention to thrive, and dotted them all over the place. They seemed to 'lift' the energy levels. I lit joss sticks to release gentle-smelling scent into the place. Fierce airsprays upset my system.

Herbal Medicine

Of all the treatments, therapies and techniques that I have tried, I consider herbal medicine to be the most effective and appropriate for my condition; a major reason for this, I am sure, was/is due to the fact that the herbalist, Mr W, is a caring, empathic, powerful healer.

During the first two to three months of treatment I attended the clinic monthly; this was to allow Mr W to monitor my progress and amend the mixture accordingly. He had tailormade a bottle of medicine for me at the first consultation.

Subsequent appointments were made every three months or so. During this time, Mr W was able to give me advice on dietary matters, general health information, and tips and guidance on managing my ME on a daily basis. He was also available via the phone if I encountered any problems, had questions, or just needed a five-minute 'pep' chat. This facility was invaluable to me; I no longer felt alone or isolated.

During the first three months of treatment the medication appeared to make the symptoms considerably more severe; however, the herbalist had mentioned that this would tend to occur, and to view it as a positive sign of healing. Herbal medicine works gently and slowly. It corrects the condition causally, rather than symptomatically.

Six months into the treatment I could not believe how much better I felt – more energised and alert; it was terrific to feel almost part of the human race again. Mr W treated me for just over a year, by which time I felt that I was well on the way to recovery, even though it was another six months before I achieved my optimum level of good health. My eyes were still very sensitive, but this was about the only remaining symptom.

Spiritual Healing

Shortly after my visit to the herbalist, I discovered Tony, a spiritual healer; by profession he was an astrologer, but I sensed that his first love was healing. He gave me weekly healing sessions, lasting some 30–35 minutes. There was no 'miracle' cure, but the positive effects built up in my system. I felt a sense of peace and calm that grew and grew. You do not require any strong religious/ spiritual belief for this kind of healing to 'work', although an open mind is helpful.

I Reshaped My Perceptions of Myself and My Illness

The most valuable thing that I was able to do for myself was to adjust the inner image of myself and my illness. I have since learned this is a technique commonly used in hypnosis; though I was not aware of it before, intuitively I felt that it would help me to recover.

I stopped seeing my condition as a punishment, or something negative, and regarded it as a friendly messenger, sent to prevent me from doing myself any further harm – indeed, to guide me on to a new pathway! (You wouldn't shoot a friendly messenger, warning of deadly danger, would you? You would embrace him/her.) I tuned into my body whenever possible. For the first time in many years I began to respect it on a health basis: I fed myself wholesome food and I began to nurture myself in many ways. I was no longer available to sort out other people's chaos, I was here for *me*!

I did not need any approval or permission to value myself; I was able to do so. My most valuable commodities now were time, love and energy. I intended to derive something very positive from this life-altering experience; if not, then I would be a victim twice over.

ME: A Process of Discovery

Rebecca Shtasel

'Illness is a great teacher,' I am sure someone once said, and so I have found ME to be.

I have been ill for three and a half years and the first year and a half was the most terrifying experience of my life. Before I became ill I had a full-time job, I went out six or seven nights a week and I firmly believed the cliché that you are only young once and should live life to the full. I tried to cram everything into my life and used the frequent viruses I got as times to rest rather than as warnings to slow down. Then one day the virus came again and this time the symptoms did not leave. I was plunged into the nightmare ME world of good days and bad days, relapses and remissions and the overwhelming sensation of being exhausted right to my inner core.

It all felt so unfair. Weren't we always being instructed to 'live each day as if it were your last'? I had tried to obey this and my reward was to become chronically ill. I felt like I was being punished; as soon as I felt well enough to go back to work or to see some friends I would relapse and be back lying exhausted and sore in my bed. My life felt completely out of control.

And yet now looking back on that time after a slow period of recovery I realise that somehow I managed to hold on and find the strength to survive. Moreover, at the same time I managed to learn that in the midst of a seeming nightmare good things do happen. ME has brought terrifyingly unexpected relapses in health and at the same time wonderfully unexpected discoveries.

I have learned how great my parents are! They thought I had left home for good and they could enjoy their retirement in peace. But no! I get ill, I return home and once again I am completely dependent on them. And they feed me and look after me and love me.

I am learning about friendship. Before I was ill friends were people to go out with. I did not really think of them as individuals with their own thoughts and ways of seeing the world. And I assumed they would stick by me no matter what. Since being ill many of them have stuck by me and some have not, including the woman I thought was my best friend. This left me very bitter, but I have now learned to see her as an individual with her own concerns which precluded me and my illness. ME has shown me the surprising qualities in my friends. Like the childhood friend with whom I had almost lost touch who began to ring regularly to see how I was, and the man with whom I had had a casual relationship who turned out to be understanding and supportive and is now a much valued friend. I have also, since being ill, met and made friends with other people who have ME. These friendships have quickly involved a level of support and intimacy born out of a shared understanding of our illness which ordinarily would take months or years or perhaps never to develop.

I have learned that I have a body which needs to be looked after. Before, my body was just a vehicle for my head, there to take me to all the places my mind wanted to go. I have learned to listen to my body; to respect its limitations. I now ask it several times a day how it is feeling and when it says it is tired I pay attention. I also regularly praise my body for coping with the onslaught of illness.

I am learning to be disciplined. Previously I had had no understanding of the meaning or the importance of discipline. But managing this illness owes a great deal to being disciplined: keeping to a routine; doing the same amount every day regardless of whether it is a good day or a bad. I have learned also to be disciplined in carrying out the activities that will improve my health. I practise every day: yoga positions, breathing exercises, meditation and relaxation. And through learning self-discipline I have learned the true meaning of control. I thought I had lost control over my life but really I had learned the hard lesson that our lives do not always go to plan. The important thing I have learned is to look after, to be kind to and to love myself because the feeling of security that gives me will enable me to survive this illness and whatever else my life has in store for me.

I am learning to have an open mind. Every day I lie on the floor with my legs up a wall and chant and this does not strike me as an odd thing to do! I have even spent time sitting in a cupboard with a large bowl of cold sugared tea and what is called a kombucha fungus in order to make a fermented drink that will supposedly cure me of my illness. And again this had seemed to me something quite normal!

I have learned that life can be exciting at any level. Excitement is found not only in activities like climbing Mount Everest or sailing the world single-handed. One of the most exciting days of my life came last year when I went by myself to the chemist and bought my own shampoo. I had not entered a shop in a year and the feeling of independence in choosing something for myself was exhilarating. I now find so many things exciting – getting a letter, doing a crossword, going to a café. Before I was ill I had such a low boredom threshold. Now, despite the fears illness brings, I can say that I enjoy so many more things than I used to.

And finally, I have learned to sit still. When I was housebound I would sit by the window and watch the cars and the people and the boats on the sea. When I could sit outside I watched the pigeons in the square. I noticed the way they walked, the way they flew, the way they courted. My head was often too foggy to think but I enjoyed looking at everything that had previously been too familiar to notice. My health has slowly improved since then (although I still have a long way to go) but I still enjoy sitting and looking. My head is clearer now and I spend time pondering so many subjects I had never considered before – the changes in the seasons, the refraction of light, the nature of colour, the workings of the mind. I have learned that 'living life to the full' does not necessarily mean running around incessantly cramming in as many experiences as possible. I live a full life now and yet I do so much less than I used to. ME has taken so much away from me and yet through having it I have learned so much that has made my life richer.

Peach, Sandalwood, Snow

Rita Wilcock

Peach, sandalwood, snow.
The snow was a surprise.

Letters nor written . . .
Ignore the lists . . .
Peaceful bath in dull winter daylight –
no piercing electric light.

Peach, sandalwood, snow.
Toys to clear away or leave –
I left them.
Across the gardens in the semi-dark
Precarious on slimy mud and slippery grass.

Still sick and tired – but there's
some peace – tranquillity in it,
A peach, sandalwood bath
in dull winter daylight.

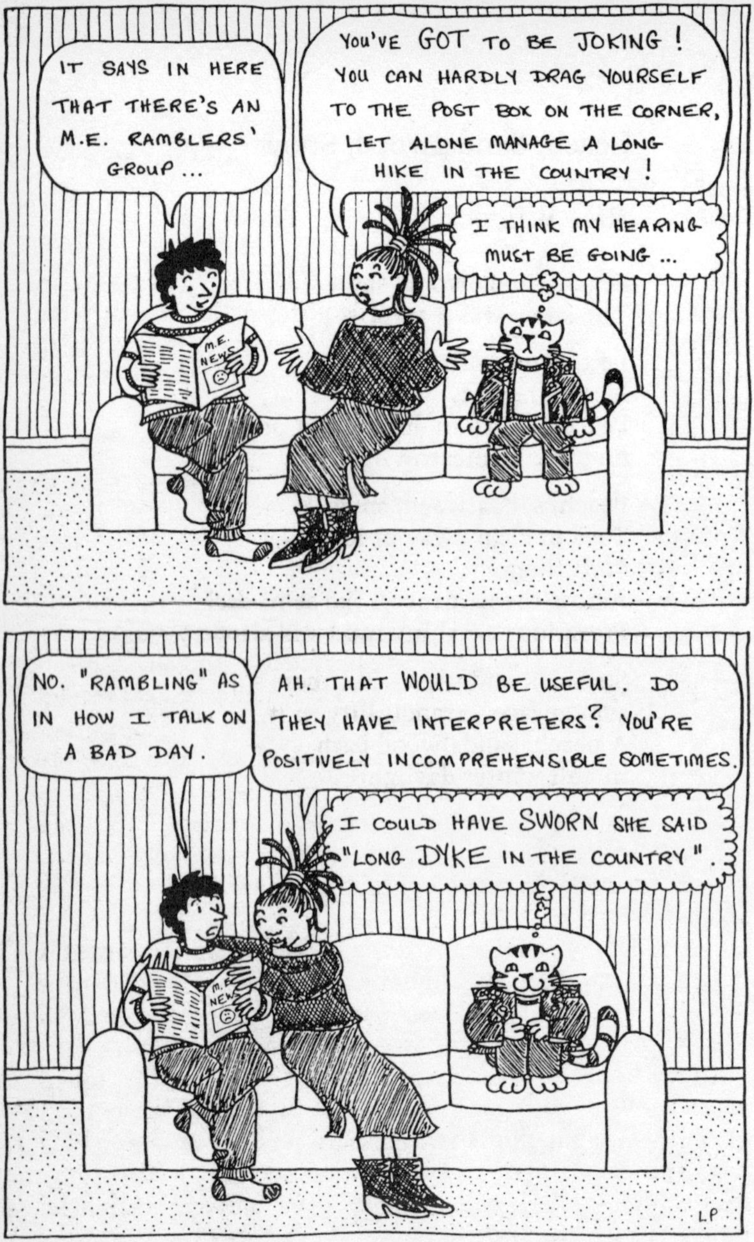
IT SAYS IN HERE THAT THERE'S AN M.E. RAMBLERS' GROUP ...
YOU'VE GOT TO BE JOKING! YOU CAN HARDLY DRAG YOURSELF TO THE POST BOX ON THE CORNER, LET ALONE MANAGE A LONG HIKE IN THE COUNTRY!
I THINK MY HEARING MUST BE GOING ...
M.E. NEWS
NO. "RAMBLING" AS IN HOW I TALK ON A BAD DAY.
AH. THAT WOULD BE USEFUL. DO THEY HAVE INTERPRETERS? YOU'RE POSITIVELY INCOMPREHENSIBLE SOMETIMES.
I COULD HAVE SWORN SHE SAID "LONG DYKE IN THE COUNTRY".
M.E. NEWS
LP

How Did I Do It?

Cordelia Galgut

I'm not quite sure when I got ME, but I was diagnosed in October 1992. I link the really debilitating form of it with getting flu in early 1990 from which I never really recovered. The final blow was an extremely bad bout of gastroenteritis which I had in the summer of 1991. After that I was laid up for 18 months, so weak I could hardly move and with a cotton wool brain. People's words sounded jumbled up – a kind of word salad that made no sense to me. I felt exasperated, desperate, very low and ill and terrified that I'd remain like this forever.

It's now almost the end of 1996, and I'm delighted and relieved to say that I have just successfully completed a very intensive and demanding two-year-long Diploma in Counselling. Five years ago I couldn't get up and make a cup of tea, let alone contemplate a re-training programme. Two and a half years on from there, I was, mainly through giving way to the illness, sleeping, sleeping and more sleeping, feeling significantly better; I'd stopped beating up on myself so much and telling myself there was nothing wrong with me; I'd been diagnosed by an ME specialist, all of which lifted my spirits and helped me to start to heal.

However, at the point that I made the decision to retrain, I was in no way well. I'm still not. Days continue to be more or less of a struggle; I still haven't got anything like the energy I used to have before ME really set in. So how did I do it?

To start with, I was fortunate that I'd been a teacher for 16 years and was retired on the basis of ill health. The process of accepting that this was necessary for me was incredibly hard and painful, but at least I came out of it with a lump sum and a small pension, which gave me some financial independence and security.

I'd heard of a foundation course in counselling skills and personal development. It happened during the day, for two hours. This would be a chance to see what I could manage. I checked out that I could lie down and cut out during the two hours, if I needed to. I was very lacking in confidence and feared I wouldn't manage.

At the time, driving was a precarious business for me; my spatial awareness wasn't so hot, nor my concentration. Also, the walk from the car park to the university was an effort in itself. I was often exhausted when I arrived. I remember always being totally spent after those two hours, hardly having the energy to walk back to the car. I used to stop in a café before driving home and indulge myself, celebrate what I'd achieved and also refuel a bit, ready for the journey home.

I would get really upset with myself at this time that my brain often wouldn't manage to process people's words – equally so on the course. I wanted to be there 100% and hated that I wasn't, that I couldn't concentrate well enough. As the course progressed, I eased up on myself in this respect. I also didn't bother with the reading – my eyes blurred if I tried to focus for more than a short while, so it would have been an ordeal anyway and I knew I couldn't manage it and the course. All I did was the journal, which was quite therapeutic. I just did a short entry each week and that sufficed. Other than the journal, there was no written work requirement. I don't think I could have managed at this point if there had been.

That foundation course, and completing it successfully, helped me regain enough confidence to enable me to go for applying for the diploma. It was an enormous risk because it was an extremely popular course, but I'm glad I took it, because it paid off and I got a place, which again boosted my belief in myself tremendously. I remember being really nervous that I wouldn't cope with the interview for it, that my body and brain wouldn't hold up. It helped that I'd said in my application that I had ME and had written about some of my processing around that. That took some pressure off me.

There was quite a long gap between the end of the

foundation course and the start of the diploma. This allowed me to rest, which helped me cope with the onslaught of the start of the diploma. The course was from 2.30 to 8.30 once a week. I'm sure I couldn't have done it if I'd been working at something else. It had to be my main focus and it was very hard, a real struggle, I can't deny that, but also enormously worthwhile and validating for me.

Often, as the day wore on, most of what was going on washed over me and I felt so exhausted I could hardly speak, and very inadequate and frustrated by my state. There were times when I should have gone home, but I was determined to have 100% attendance for my own reasons, although the course demanded 80%. Psychologically, I wanted the 100%, almost as though getting it would be proof I was better. I was also thinking of future job applications and how 100% attendance might counterbalance my poor attendance record when I was ill before I retired. Even though pushing myself was very expensive for me, because I had several relapses during the course which made me feel lousy, physically and emotionally, as well as having no energy for anything but the course, I'm still glad I went for it.

Overall, course members and tutors were ME friendly. I took the opportunity at times to talk about my feelings about my illness, and I think this helped them understand. For example, on one occasion I remember telling the group that I was really scared about an imminent residential weekend because I didn't think I'd be able to keep going. It was hard for me to do this and admit to weakness as I saw it, but it paid off because at the weekend people were really supportive. In a sense, it was me who was my own worst enemy during the weekend. People encouraged me to lie down far more than I actually did. I hated to miss out on anything. That's me. On one of the course weekends, I did withdraw to rest and that felt fine and helped me get through the time more easily. There's no denying, though, that I felt better able to because I felt safer and more secure in the group by then.

There were many occasions throughout the course when the constant contact with people was so exhausting that I just couldn't manage any more and I cut out in a variety of ways, because I had to. Sometimes, I would just sit and nod and not be there. Other times, I would go and lie down somewhere. I'd tell myself I'd done enough and I'd earned it and that seemed to work for me.

Written work was enjoyable and hard. I worked and re-worked things in an unnecessarily perfectionist way. I could have passed the course without doing this. I know, though, that doing so was part of my processing around ME. I was proving to myself that I had the energy to stick with my thoughts and feelings and explore them unrelentingly, until I was satisfied. That was such an achievement for me and a sign I was so much better. Overall I didn't read anything like as much as I should have or wanted to and I regret this, but that's how I survived. Staying in touch with my feelings was important, being aware of when I felt overwhelmed; allowing myself to feel that. Sleeping a lot helped and having days on a regular basis when I allowed myself to forget about the work. A course requirement was to complete 100 hours of client work. I managed this by starting it as soon as I could and spreading it out in a manageable way, so that at the end of the course I wasn't panicking about it.

At the start of the course, I felt really deskilled, having lost my job and not worked for a while. By the end of it, I felt much better, much more hopeful about my future and enormously empowered.

Yes, I've got ME and might well have forever. But I now have a new career. I feel tons better for it psychologically and no worse physically. Where to go from here isn't clear and a real worry, given that I'm still quite disabled by my illness, but I've definitely got more choices now. I did push myself a lot, when perhaps I shouldn't have, because it made my ME worse. For me, the important thing then was to recognise what was happening to me and stop, no matter what. This is, and continues to be, so hard for me – how to achieve the right balance of doing and stopping. But I did manage to pull back enough and rest enough to get myself through the course and that was the main thing in the end!

The Battle for Life

Amanda Cornu

My last drop of blood
is lost
to some unknown enemy
Shed on a battlefield
of pain and total exhaustion
Days are long
I drag myself about
brandishing my weapon
fighting as I can
But my wounds are too deep
Healing impossible
The day has been
just too long
The enemy overwhelming
Will-power not sufficient
Soldiering on
No longer possible
the day's ending
approaches
As a sun sets splendidly
My body aches
in every limb
My head and neck
a barrage of knives
My legs will barely carry me
But my eyes are intact
The setting sun enticing
Its beauty resplendent
and life worth living.

Fantasies, Realities and a Bit of Common Sense

Elina Rigler

A Magical Theory of Holism

I sometimes feel that the worst aspect of having a chronic illness is not living with the limitations it places on my life, but putting up with the myths surrounding it. One of the myths I've been puzzling over recently is that of 'illness personality'. It seems to pop up everywhere: both scientific and religious experts claim that it is one of the factors that contribute to illnesses like ME.

Until quite recently most mainstream doctors took a rather mechanistic view of disease. They assumed that physical illnesses had a single external cause, which could be identified by laboratory tests and treated by drugs or surgery. These days the majority of health professionals, including those practising conventional medicine, hold the view that illnesses have multiple causes. Not only do they take account of microbes, but also factors like pollution, poor diet, psychological and social stress, and the more religiously-minded even talk about spiritual imbalance. They attempt to treat the 'real' cause of illness, and not just symptoms, and are, therefore, willing to prescribe complementary therapies and recommend psychological counselling. Today a so-called holistic approach to treatment is so widely accepted that it can no longer be called alternative.

Many people will welcome the new holistic approach to health. They are dissatisfied with the outdated scientific view of illness, which ignores the wholeness of the person. They want to be treated as individuals with emotional, social and spiritual needs, not as machines with broken parts. Adopting a healthier lifestyle, reducing stress and other holistic approaches to health are, of course, just common sense. The trouble is that the pendulum has swung so far the other way that many people now accept the holistic philosophy uncritically. By focusing too closely on the power of mind we are in danger of distorting reality and creating fantasies. The simple idea that body and mind are inextricably linked seems to have developed into a magical theory of holism.

So I'm concerned about the fact that one set of dogmatic beliefs has been replaced by another. I think there are a number of questions that are not being asked, and new truths that are not being challenged within the holistic approach. One such truth is that most illness is stress-induced. The interesting question is that if stress is present everywhere in modern life, and all of us suffer from it most of the time, why is it that some people get ill and not others? This is where the notion of 'illness personality' comes in, providing the missing link in the chain. It becomes the Factor X that can be used to explain why some people are unable to withstand stress, and as a result fall ill, and even worse, fail to recover.

Illness Personality – General Characteristics

There is an ever-expanding junk literature of illness, which offers some extremely nutty accounts of emotional or spiritual causes of illnesses. Louise Hay, the Barbara Cartland of illness books, has produced some of the nuttiest ones. She thinks that there is a link between people's emotional states on the one hand and *specific* illnesses on the other.[1] According to her, asthma can be linked to 'fear of life' and vaginal infections to 'sexual guilt'. As one reviewer has pointed out, in Hay's world bodies are not only 'embarrassingly Freudian' but also 'wicked punmakers': bladder problems, for instance, result from being 'pissed off', and polio from 'paralyzing jealousy'.[2]

Bernie Siegel is another guru with a large following who also likes word games.[3] His patients get breast cancer because they show a negative attitude towards their breasts, or leukaemia because they hold their feelings inside. Those unfortunate souls who avoid emotional growth run the risk of developing a malignant physical growth. These sorts of books are full of stereotypical heroic people who overcome their fear of life and recover miraculously by sending love into their tumours and welcome suffering with open arms because it provides a wonderful opportunity for emotional and spiritual growth.

Most people are able to treat these kinds of books with the same degree of cynicism as any other products of junk culture. Matching up emotional states with physical illnesses is a bit of fun – a parlour game we can all play on a rainy day. These books have the nutritional value of candy floss, but they are fairly harmless unless you mistake them for a proper meal. If, like me, you are allergic to sugar, reading sentences like 'She chose the path of life, and as she grew, her cancer shrank'[4] can do funny things to your system.

We get into difficulties when we mistake these word games for reality; when we start believing that people really do get ill because they avoid spiritual growth. It's important to remember that they are *not* scientific theories, neither are they God-given truths. They're only fairy tales, and have the same tenuous connection with real life as soap operas or Hollywood movies. What Louise Hay, Bernie Siegel and Co. offer you is not profound wisdom, but pop spirituality at its very worst. It's definitely time to take a reality check when you catch yourself suggesting that you got ill because of your relationship with your mother, or that so and so's negative attitude has delayed her recovery.

Not all books that mention 'illness personality' are quite this barmy; however, I still have reservations about most of them. Many of them refer to the familiar Type A personality, who is 'competitive', 'hostile', and 'accomplishment-orientated', and therefore prone to heart disease. Another often-mentioned personality type is the Type C, who is said to be 'passive', 'over-sensitive', and 'emotionally repressed', and likely to get cancer, and sometimes also arthritis.[5] There is also an increasing number of spiritual books which identify 'deep' causes of physical disease, such as 'a deep feeling of emptiness' and 'deep imbalances'.[6] (We could call those suffering from spiritual problems 'Type S' people.)

The problem is that these descriptions are so general that they can apply to most people – is there anyone who hasn't behaved competitively or repressed her emotions at times? Vague spiritual descriptions, such as 'inner emptiness' and 'lack of harmony', are especially handy because they fit every person and every complaint. It seems to me that since human beings are by definition spiritually flawed, all of us can be said to be Type S personalities. Worse still, the same illness is sometimes associated with two conflicting character flaws. For instance, some books portray cancer sufferers as being too dependent, and others as too independent.[7] (This latter description naturally applies mainly to women. There is nothing more disturbing than an independent woman – illness is an appropriate punishment for her.) The details don't seem all that important; the sick person is simply 'too something or other'. She has become ill and refuses to get better, so she must have a personality disorder.

Quite a few authors seek support from scientific research for their mind-body theories. (Interestingly enough, these authors include those with New Agey leanings, who normally pour scorn on anything as rational as scientific activity.) For instance, Marc Ian Barasch, who seems very keen on the notion of illness personality, refers to a number of studies showing a link between emotional repression and cancer.[8] What I'd like to know is how is it possible to measure 'disorders' such as emotional repression, without reducing the complexity of an individual's behaviour to a handful of psychological clichés? In any case, all of us need to suppress our emotions most of the time – only babies and toddlers and the filthy rich are free to vent their frustration without being ostracised from civilised society. When is the suppression of emotions appropriate, when is it pathological, and who decides which is which?

Another question that has been puzzling me for quite some time is how exactly emotions, or lack of them, 'cause' illness? To take one example, someone suffering an emotional trauma, say, bereavement, might get ill because she is too distressed to look after herself. She might stop taking her medication, sleep badly, and forget to eat properly. This is a plausible explanation, but sounds rather banal. It's therefore less attractive than the romantic idea that it's the suppressed passions or unexpressed grief that mysteriously develop into a tumour, because they have nowhere else to go.

Incidentally, who stands to gain most from these simplistic ideas about illness personality? The psychologists, who boost their careers (and egos) by identifying yet another personality type/psychological disorder? The New Age gurus, who make money out of popularising 'scientific' theories? The family and friends of the patient, who can take comfort from the fact that only Type X people get ill? Definitely not the patient, who feels guilty about being such a pathetic failure at the game of life, and who worries that she might never recover unless she transforms her personality.

Many people don't feel the need to ask these sorts of questions. It's far easier to give in to intellectual laziness and parrot the 'truth' that emotional repression causes disease. We forget that research findings are often a good deal less clear-cut than most of us would care to think. For instance, it is common knowledge that stress suppresses the immune function and makes us susceptible to disease. The fact is, though, that many scientific experts treat findings in this field with more caution than lay people. They are only too aware of the complexity of the immune system, and are unwilling to make irresponsible generalisations about the link between emotional stress and disease. I was interested to read recently the following statement by a biologist and a neuroscientist: 'Although evidence is emerging that stress-induced immunosuppression can indeed increase the risk and severity of disease, the connection is probably relatively weak and its importance is often exaggerated'.[9] A view like this is so commonsensical that it fails to grab your attention. Most people will probably ignore it altogether, especially since the author goes on to say that there is no scientific evidence at present to support the claim that we can heal ourselves through positive thinking.

I find it fascinating to look at these issues from a historical point of view. One interesting fact is that the meaning we give to illnesses changes over time and reflects the medical advances and psychological theories of the day.[10] (It's not surprising that at a time when self-expression and the pursuit of happiness are all but compulsory, emotional repression rather than, say, lack of compassion is a serious flaw.) For instance, before the medical causes of TB were understood, it was regarded as a romantic disease of excessive passion, which affected love-sick maidens and hypersensitive artists. Today TB has lost its glamour: most of us think of it as a rather mundane disease and associate it mainly with poverty and poor hygiene.

It also seems to me that it is only when we cannot link a disease to poverty or malnutrition that we need to look for a 'deeper' explanation – an illness personality is a luxury that only well-fed people living in nice houses can enjoy. I didn't see any references to 'cholera personality' ('a person with such low self-esteem that she chooses to live in poverty'?) during recent cholera epidemics in India. It would be equally obscene to suggest that those amongst the homeless who suffer from 'inner emptiness' develop TB, when this emptiness might simply mean that they haven't eaten for several days.

The truth is that nobody knows what the truth is. All we have is a collection of theories about the possible link between emotional states and illness, which often say more about their authors than about the phenomena they are meant to explain. It's probably true that major and prolonged emotional stress increases the *risk* of disease, which is not the same as saying that stress 'causes' disease, or that only 'emotionally repressed' people get ill. It's also one thing to say that self-help techniques may contribute to the healing process, and quite another to claim that we can control our immune function by practising meditation and visualisation and positive thinking. The sad thing is that in the guise of encouraging 'self-empowerment', 'positivity' and 'self-responsibility', many authors of self-help books promote unrealistic, and even moralistic, ideas about health. In particular, their readers are led to believe in the following two fantasies: first, you will not fall ill if you deal with stress in a healthy manner (whatever 'healthy' means in this context); and second, you can overcome your illness by expressing your inner needs and having enough hope and courage.

ME Personality

Like other poorly understood illnesses, ME is surrounded by myths and fantasies. Religious and scientific experts both resort to magic to fill in the gaps in their knowledge.

In New Agey books people suffering from ME are presented as a subtype of the Type S personality. According to a healer, Nick Bamforth, ME strikes people who have suppressed their creative life force, and as a result suffer from 'inner emptiness'. In Bamforth's words, 'The gulf between one's inner aspirations and the outer mask is not just symbolic; as this gulf becomes wider, a very real and ever growing emptiness develops between them, a void which allows a consciousness such as cancer, ME or any major disease to enter within.'[11] (Beautiful, isn't it? Who needs logic or reality when you can have this sentimental tosh? Then again, only spiritually impoverished people like me let facts get in the way of a good theory.) 'Imbalance' is another common problem. Bamforth claims that especially women with ME often suffer from 'imbalance between the male and female', which manifests 'as a predominance of the male, assertive, rational, side of human nature over the more female, nurturing, intuitive side.'[12] (So that's where I went wrong. I made the wrong career choice – I should have become an Earth Mother. Where have I heard this reactionary claptrap before? Oh yeah, it was some politician banging on about working mothers and family values.) After carefully listing all the spiritual flaws of people with ME, Bamforth tells us that we shouldn't feel guilty and ought never to judge ourselves, because there're no 'shoulds' and 'oughts'. (What did I just say about logic?) I disagree: anyone who writes for public consumption sentences like 'Guilt, by smothering your life force, can literally kill'[13] ought to feel very guilty indeed!

And this is the gospel of New Age: You can take control of your life and heal yourself if you work hard and stop running away from your True Self. Get in touch with your spiritual side, love yourself, let go of anger and go beyond fear. Above all, become balanced and fill that inner void with Beauty and Truth and Love. If you don't recover after all this it is because deep down you want to be ill; you will recover when you have no further need for your illness. Your need to be ill – this is the missing Factor X that explains why some people 'choose the path of life' while others resist change and remain ill.

This stuff should carry a health warning: it is likely to raise your blood pressure and leave you feeling nauseous. It's only recommended for those with a strong stomach and a peculiar sense of humour.

Many 'secular' self-help books on ME, including those written by 'respectable' medical professionals, also devote some space to the notion of ME personality. In Belinda Dawes' and Damien Downing's experience, almost all people with ME are 'goal-orientated' and 'strive hard to gain recognition and approval' because they suffer from a 'deep-seated lack of self-acceptance'.[14] These sorts of personality defects and attitudes give rise to 'illness behaviour'. Driven by their pathological need to reach their goals, some people rush back to work before they have fully recovered from an infection. This is how they develop a chronic form of ME.

The above description manages to combine neatly the

Type A and Type C personalities: ME sufferers are stubborn and goal-orientated, as well as being meek and dependent. Again, one might point out that descriptions such as 'goal-orientated' or 'seeking recognition' fit most people most of the time. They can, in fact, apply to any 'normal' adult living in modern Western society, where business and achievement are considered to be virtues. (Ironically, those who preach the gospel of 'being, not doing' are always extremely busy themselves writing books and giving talks on this very subject.) The difference is, of course, that healthy people don't suffer from a lack of self-acceptance, at least not from a *deep-seated* lack. It's the Factor X again, always capable of distinguishing the sick from the healthy.

It's probably true that the vast majority of ME sufferers do fail to take appropriate care during the initial stages of the illness. However, there might be reasons for this behaviour, other than a desperate need for approval. Some of them may be economic. You may crawl out of bed and go to work too early because of a deep-seated financial insecurity. Of course, being broke is much less interesting an explanation for 'illness behaviour' than a psycho-spiritual one, such as lack of self-love. What Dawes and Downing seem to ignore is that fighting illness, rather than giving in to it, is the culturally acceptable form of behaviour. When you fail to recover, your family and friends, your employer, and even your doctor may put pressure on you to stop playing the invalid, instead of encouraging you to rest. Another rather obvious point is that since being seriously ill may be a completely new experience for you, you're likely to make mistakes in the early stages of the illness. It can take months or years to work out what's good for your body and mind, and even then, because of the peculiarity and variability of the symptoms, you keep getting it wrong.

There is a competing view of the ME personality, which is popular amongst psychiatrists and other influential medical professionals. According to this view, it is *avoidance* of activity that leads to a chronic form of 'ME'.[15] Apparently, some deluded people believe that they're ill and therefore indulge in 'illness behaviour'. They stop going out and stay in bed, with the result that they get out of condition and feel depressed. The good news is that there is a cure for this 'illness'. First you need to stop thinking that you're ill, then you take a quick stroll round the park, followed by a nice cup of tea, and you'll be well on your way to recovery. (The technical term for this type of treatment is 'cognitive behaviour therapy' (CBT).)

You really cannot win if you have ME: whatever you do, someone will wag an accusing finger at you. Some people treat ME sufferers as depressed and apathetic Type C personalities ('Come on, a little exercise will do you good!'), others as hyperactive Type A personalities ('No wonder you're ill – you never stop, do you?'). Sufferers themselves can play this game. When I have done something that's knocked me out, I often tell myself: 'Oh it's my ME personality'. What I really mean is that I'm not a saint, and I make mistakes. I didn't realise that doing X would make me worse, or I suspected that it might, but I did it anyway because I needed to get out of the house. It is impossible to be ill month in, month out, year after year, and never do anything naughty. ('Naughty' is the *mot juste* here. You can almost feel the raps on your knuckles when you've broken School Mistress Dawes' 75 per cent rule.[16])

Your doctor may not be a follower of Louise Hay and Bernie Siegel, but she probably knows all about 'psycho-social stress' and 'masked depression'. As she cannot offer you any conventional treatment, she may well try to treat you 'holistically'. In practice this often means a referral to a psychiatrist or a cognitive behaviour therapist. You'd be mad to admit to your doctor that you might occasionally feel depressed or anxious when she is apt to translate an ordinary human experience (a reaction to a difficult situation) into Medicalese ('depressive illness' and 'anxiety disorder'). It's hard to imagine a normally functioning human being who wouldn't, once in a while, experience anxiety and even despair when faced with a serious chronic illness. Try explaining this to someone who, because of her faith in holism, equates chronic illness with personality disorder.

Counsellors and alternative therapists may also be eager to distract your attention from the reality of your situation, and explore your childhood traumas and psychological helplessness – the 'true' causes of your illness. You might seek emotional support, but what you often get is 'treatment' for your deep-seated psychological problems. If you so much as hint that your life is less than perfect you may be subjected to a barrage of therapeutic clichés and intrusive interpretations. (This is even more likely to happen if you've failed to live up to the cultural ideals of womanhood, e.g. if you're not wife and mother.) There is little emphasis on the positive aspects of your life; on the fact that you are coping, however imperfectly. Some health professionals cannot accept the fact that you're an intelligent adult, and the only true expert on your mental and physical health. I find it ironic that those who advise you to take control of your life and trust your intuition often get exceedingly annoyed when you do precisely that by resisting their authority.

Work and achievement are a natural part of adult life and an important source of personal satisfaction. Losing the ability to do things is a heavy blow to anyone; wanting to be active is healthy, not a sign of illness personality. 'Being' is lovely, but only if you can mix it with 'doing'. I've always been struck by how well-adjusted people with ME are, even those who are severely affected. Despite all the losses they've suffered, they have managed to find creative solutions to the problems of living with a chronic illness. This is another fact that the illness literature fails to emphasise.

Fantasy World vs Real World

It's occurred to me that both scientific and religious 'experts' have a curiously sanitised view of human life. They seem to be living in a Fantasy World where perfectly adjusted people without negative thoughts go through life in neat stages, or

– to use spiritual jargon – 'true selves' live in harmony and love each other unconditionally, letting go of anger and fear. This is also a just world. The psychosocially or spiritually adequate people (aka the 'Whole People'[17]) glow with health and cosmic love (and, incidentally, make pots of money), whilst the inadequate ones (Types A, C, S, and ME) are condemned to chronic illness and poverty. The sick can be saved and become Whole People if they repent and change their ways - but if you lead an averagely unhappy life, you can forget about salvation.

In the Fantasy World there's an answer for every question, a solution to every problem. The experts have solved the mysteries of Life and the Universe and the Deep Causes of Chronic Illness. 'It's depression', some of them will tell us with absolute conviction, while others blame it on 'stress', 'illness beliefs', or 'fear of life'. Above all, it is within our control and treatable. The sick can be restored to perfect balance, or at least to 'normality', through psychotherapy, graded exercise, alternative medicine, emotional expression or relaxation techniques. While advising the sick to fight fear, the gurus themselves are so afraid of looking reality in the face that they hide behind all-purpose theories and spiritual babble. We all do this, 'experts' and 'lay people', the sick and the healthy alike. We make up comforting stories about the meaning of mental and physical pain, longing for the security of the Fantasy World. As author and psychologist Ken Wilber points out, people have always searched for a simple cause for suffering as 'a natural and understandable defence against the fear of the unknown'.[18]

What we need is humility to accept that some things are beyond our control, and – contrary to popular belief - there is no cure for the human condition. Human life is full of pain; perfect love and perfect harmony are but fantasies; some issues will always remain unresolved; and our relations with one another will never be free of conflict. The Whole Person with her secure sense of self and inner harmony is just another myth – a myth created by those who're so busy mouthing platitudes that they wouldn't recognise a real person even if she came along and hit them with a copy of *You Can Heal Your Life*. Real people experience real emotions, sometimes even fear and envy and anger. They muddle through life, going round in circles and making mistakes over and over again.

In the Real World, illness has no meaning; it's just 'life'. The sick person is neither a victim (an inadequate personality who needs to be 'normalised' or 'harmonised'), nor a romantic heroine who faces adversity with a beatific smile on her face. She is just an ordinary person trying to cope the best she can in difficult circumstances. No one living in the Real World can avoid pain, conflict, confusion, uncertainty, or even 'inner emptiness'. Real life is frequently hard and frustrating, but also infinitely more mysterious than life in the Fantasy World.

Common Sense, My Best Friend

I'd like to put in a plea for common sense, which seems to be in short supply in recent illness literature. I use common sense to guide me when I wade through the ME literature, pore over statistics, and weigh up the benefits of various treatments and diets. It tells me I'd be foolish not to take responsibility for my health and make the necessary changes to my lifestyle; it's undoubtedly better for me to be relaxed and think positively than to be tense and miserable. However, it also tells me that it's not always possible to remain calm and optimistic and, moreover, that it's not within my power to cure myself by changing my lifestyle, expressing my 'inner needs' and thinking beautiful thoughts. I realise that common sense isn't nearly as exciting as magic, but I value my sanity more than the cheap thrills available to the inhabitants of the Fantasy World.

This is my personal affirmation: I promise to love myself enough not to read New Age trash, and every day I'll spend some time visualising a brave new world where no one talks about 'illness beliefs', 'illness behaviour' or 'illness personality'.

I'm feeling better already.

Notes

1 Hay, Louise, *You Can Heal Your Life*, Eden Grove Editions, Enfield, 1988.
2 Ince, Susan, 'Blaming the Victim', in *Savvy Woman*, cited in *Interaction* No, 9, Spring 1992.
3 Siegel, Bernie, *Love, Medicine and Miracles*, Harper and Row, New York, 1986.
4 ibid., p.113.
5 See e.g. Pelletier, Kenneth, *Mind as Healer, Mind as Slayer*, Dell, New York, 1977, and Gawler, Ian, *You Can Conquer Cancer*, Thorsons, Wellingborough, 1986.
6 Bamforth, Nick, *Aids and the Healer Within*, Amethyst Books, New York, 1993 is a typical representative of this 'genre'.
7 According to Gawler, op.cit., those prone to cancer are overly dependent, while in Ken Wilber's *Grace and Grit*, Gill & Macmillan Ltd, Dublin, 1991 they are described as being too independent.
8 Barasch, Marc Ian, *The Healing Path*, Penguin/Arkana Books, New York, 1993.
9 Sapolsky, Robert, *Why Zebras Don't Get Ulcers*, WH Freeman and Co., New York, 1994, p. 33.
10 This is discussed elegantly in Sontag Susan, *Illness as Metaphor*, Penguin Books, London, 1983.
11 Bamforth, op. cit., p. 122.
12 ibid., p. 56.
13 ibid., p. 130.
14 Dawes, Belinda, and Downing, Damien, *Why ME?*, Grafton Books, London, 1989.
15 cf. e.g. the recent report by the Medical Royal Colleges on Chronic Fatigue Syndrome (October 1996). These eminent medical professionals have banned the use of the term 'ME'. Those who think they suffer from 'ME' can only be saved by massive doses of cognitive behaviour therapy.
16 According to this rule, you should only do 75 per cent of what you can do without suffering a relapse.
17 I'm using the term 'whole person' here in the way Rosalind Coward uses it in her wonderfully perceptive *The Whole Truth – The Myth of Alternative Health* (Faber and Faber, London, 1989). It refers to this mythical being who is perfectly balanced and has no negative emotions.
18 Wilber, Ken, op.it., p. 219.

The Magic Paintbox: Art and ME

Kate Adams

My earliest memories are of colours: green, red and orange, my plastic alphabet letters; plum and purple, my sister's snake necklace; yellow, gold and ochre, the flesh of Gauguin's Tahitian women and Van Gogh's bedroom chair in the picture books my father kept.

I was six or seven when I had my first paintbox, a dark blue metal box of watercolours. I savoured the names of each small block of paint: Vandyke Brown, Viridian, Hookers Green, Crimson Lake. Mysterious names that evoked stories. I still love their sound.

As a child I drew and painted fluidly. People and horses, streets and landscapes were my favourite subjects. My paintbox gave me access to another world fired by my imagination. At Art College some of this was beaten out of me. Instinct and passion gave way to reason, rhythmic lines to angles and perspective, colour was subdued by tone. I was learning things that would make me a better painter. All the same anxiety set in. I never felt I met required standards.

Leaving college and getting a job I redefined myself as an adult, a social worker and political activist. I became responsible and took on other people's problems instead of always thinking about myself. There was little time for painting. This was partly a relief. I was able to use art in my job, so I didn't completely let go of it. In a women's group I set-up, and in work with people with learning difficulties, colours and shapes were sometimes an alternative language when verbal communication failed.

Professional employment helped my development but something was repressed, if not entirely crushed when I stopped painting – the aspect of ourselves not visible or tangible, vitality. The vital force, homeopaths call it.

When I became ill, I turned to colour again as if reunited with an absent friend. In January 1989, off sick from work and on the cusp of having ME I wrote in my journal:

'Today was flowering. It was so warm I almost took my coat off. There were birds singing all over Hackney. In the morning I went to the Stoke Newington art shop, Vortex, and bought a Post Impressionist Diary '89 with prints of Bonnard, Vuillard, Matisse, Bernard. I also bought a calendar with flowers on it and some coloured pastels.'

The purchase of the box of oil pastels mentioned almost inconsequentially was an important decision. I was both seeking a weapon to fight the illness with and beginning a new phase as an artist.

These bright crayons, reminiscent of my childhood paints, were a box of magic tricks. I could conjure visions of a place beyond the illness which threatened my mental as well as physical being. I began with drawings in a sketch book; mostly these were landscapes, views from the window of the street or of my friends' and parents' gardens. Observing what was outside and translating it into an image that was my own, compensated for being forced to stay inside.

Through looking closely at trees and plants, and the changing skies, in all kinds of weather, I have found both a healing quality and a connection with the landscape. Getting an electric wheelchair a few years ago has meant increased independence and access to the parks, the river and the marshes near my home. Drawings and colour studies of these are now the basis of larger paintings. Colour and light are essential to my work. I am now using colour more imaginatively to convey mood and emotion.

Painting has helped me survive ME and ME brought me back to painting as surely as it took away so much that I still grieve for. Eight years on I haven't quite given up on recovery. Sometimes I think that the relationship between my artwork and the natural world holds the key. At others this seems like mystical nonsense. Here is what I wrote in February 1997 after a morning drawing up on the hill in Springfield Park when the sinusitis I had been stuck with for two weeks vanished:

'I sat on the seat facing the marshes by the stiff green hedges for a bit less than two hours. My feet froze and the wind blew all my symptoms away. I did something that said what I feel about winter, the subtle colours, stark trees - I prefer them leafless or just in bud – and everything I felt about the park and the marshes came in too. So at the end I was part of the rust-coloured bushes and stick-like trees, the blue-grey river and the van parked, small like a child's toy, the scattered red, pink and lilac of receding houses, white verticles of tower blocks under a moving sky.'

This is an example of how beneficial art is when everything flows, but it happened after several months of being unwell and blocked creatively. There is still a tension between instinct and reason for me in the process of painting which I find difficult. One day I hope to paint simply and powerfully with all the joy and spontaneity of childhood: A time when pain and illness were always temporary.

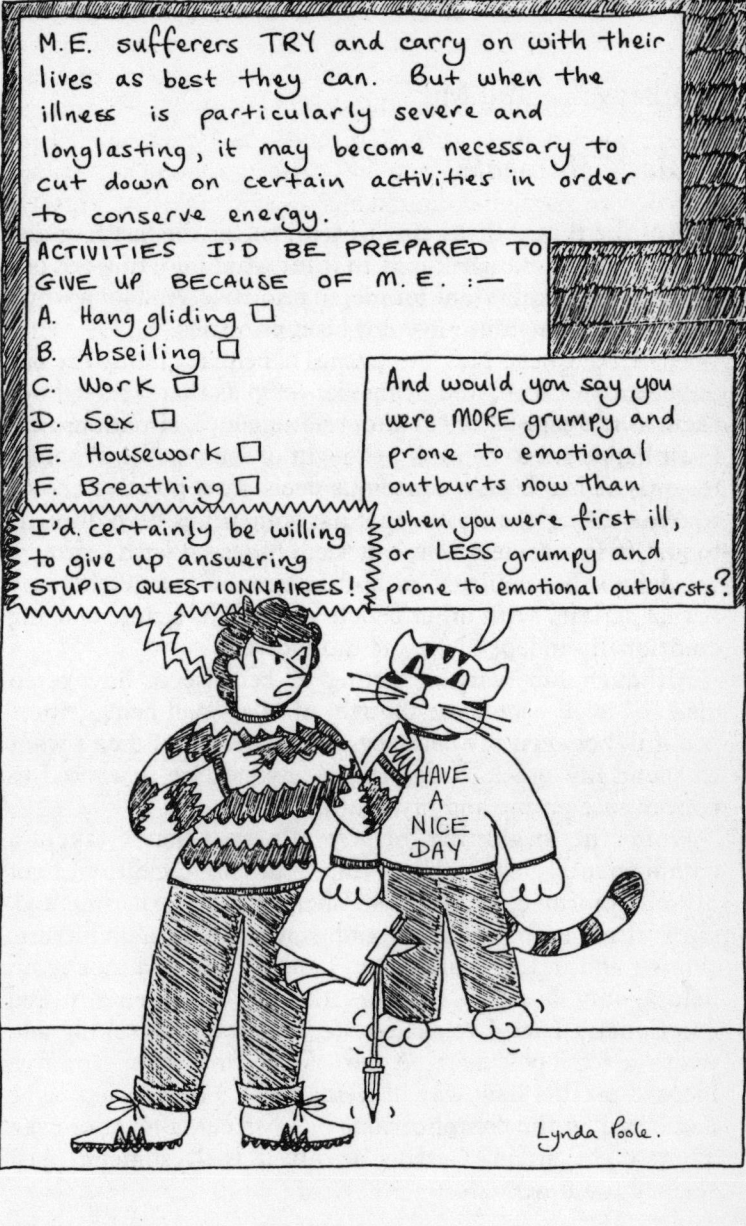

Celibacy, ME and Me

Lydia Nightingale

One of the things that being ill with ME for the last four and a half years has taught me is to limit what I do, to work out what really is important for me, to prioritise. And for a while sex and relationships have not been priorities.

There have been previous phases of celibacy in my life but only retrospectively did I consider them as that. I thought of them as the gaps before or after relationships, situations that I just happened to be in, if I thought of them at all. Whereas recently it has been a conscious decision, a positive choice to remain single; a choice that has sometimes been difficult to justify in a society that can seem obsessed with sex.

I define this celibacy as both a time of not having any sexual activity with other people and also as a time of being emotionally independent and uninvolved.

Although I'm wary of saying it, because of how often disabled or ill people are thought of as asexual beings, there *is* a link between my celibacy and ME because I didn't want to spend my precious energy on anyone else, I wanted to concentrate on me and my health.

From the beginning of my illness I have taken a complementary approach to improving my condition. I got myself informed, joined a self-help group, 'experimented' with alternative therapies and stayed with acupuncture, shiatsu and nutritional advice. I spent time and money on helping my body to recover. To help me mentally and emotionally I used relaxation techniques, counselling and wrote a log book/diary. A lot of my limited energy was focused on this new way of living and I did not want to be distracted by the complications of a partner, a lover or even a one-night stand. Getting involved with someone just seemed too much effort.

I could imagine that many practical problems could arise from having a girlfriend whilst coping with the symptoms of ME, but I could also envisage possible solutions: spending relaxed time together (reading to each other, watching films, taking short walks or drives, special meals in or out), devising 'plan B's' in case of tiredness, planning an unconventional social life or dates (around daytime/quiet/ home-based/smoke-free/less active events) and creating a sex life that accommodated symptoms such as low energy levels and sleep problems. But I couldn't imagine a solution to the level of mental and emotional involvement that's also required in relationships, whether long- or short-term. I needed freedom from that kind of responsibility.

As ME means I have had to cope with both physical and mental exhaustion, I have used some of the energy, that in the past would have gone into a relationship, on myself to sort out the issues that being ill has created for me and to find out how to live my life.

This solitude has given me space to create new, affirming rituals for myself:

- enjoying exchanging long letters with someone I care about
- being aware of the seasons as I watch my plants and herbs slowly grow
- nurturing myself by creating exciting puddings within my dietary restrictions
- learning, as an ex-hill walker, to appreciate the country- side differently and to enjoy the once-criticised activity of a car ride and sitting in a lay-by with a flask
- treating myself to the sensual pleasure of a warm bath with lavender and patchouli oils
- trying to identify the birds that visit the bird table in my garden
- listening to a radio play or my favourite music, whilst lying in bed
- enhancing my 'hot water bottle and slippers' image by learning how to knit

- getting totally absorbed in trashy novels and travel books
- indulging in long phone calls
- painting my stomach with henna and my toenails with silver or blue nail varnish
- developing a tradition of breakfast in bed whilst wearing my full-length dressing gown, and drinking herbal tea from 1960s crockery

Through having ME I have learnt to appreciate the calmer things in life, and being lover-free has given me uncluttered time to be with myself, my thoughts and my feelings.

Finding the Strength to Meet the Challenges of ME

Marcia Francis Spence

I have learned many lessons during the past year. In doing so I had to ask myself a number of questions and simultaneously find the answers within myself, for example:

1. How do I provide myself with the nourishment to repair and minimise future damage to my body?
2. How do I vocalise what has happened to me so others can take what they need from my experience?
3. How does my experience with ME fit into the rest of my life?
4. How do I fight the despair which results from the internal enemies of fear, anger and powerlessness.

I am now taking time to appreciate and enjoy life, ensuring I keep my priorities clearly in focus.

My only option has been to reach deep inside myself, identify honestly how I feel, and ascertain what it is I really want from now on and proceed to act on it.

Having made the decision, I feel comfortable with it and able to move on. I have taken the year to learn to love and appreciate myself in a different way by trying to adjust to the changes rather than resisting them.

The wider culture encourages us to view wellness as a luxury to be experienced exclusively by the white population. It is important that black people counter such a view. Validating our stories is a significant part of that process. We have a duty to acknowledge and chart our experiences from our own perspective rather than rely on others to do it for us. It is acceptable to acknowledge our pain as only by doing so can we accept it, become receptive to our own healing powers, and begin to heal. Being forced to examine my whole life critically and urgently has in fact left me stronger and in no doubt that the most important resource I have is myself.

Meeting the Challenge: Dealing with the Diagnosis

I am learning to work through the illness by living differently, and the vision of the future I can now create has been informed by the knowledge of my limitations.

Initially I harboured a feeling of insignificance and therefore wanted to isolate myself. I did not want anyone to see me in such a vulnerable state and I doubted I would recover. I had battled with the medical profession in trying to arrive at a diagnosis and spent time, energy and finances on private consultations and treatment, all of which had taken its toll, with the result that I now felt weighed down and drained.

I was a mere shadow of my former self that even I did not recognise. I could not converse with anyone on the telephone because I was very emotional and the tears were never far away. My strength had deserted me, my positive outlook also, and I did not want to be part of the world as I was unable to see a future. I could not even communicate through letters because I had difficulty constructing sentences; my handwriting was shaky; and my concentration so limited that I became embarrassed at what I managed to produce.

In my quest to move up the career ladder I had learned to operate beyond sensible limits. I had ceased to listen to my body, choosing instead to struggle on. There was only one way to begin to undo the damage and that was to listen to my body. I had to now concentrate on *being* rather than doing and so initially I became anti-social, cutting myself off from the outside world and relying on relaxation and prayer to carry me through each day.

Meeting the Challenges: Facing the Complexity of the Losses

I cried until I felt there were no tears left, but even if I had cried for a hundred years I could not possibly have expressed the sorrow I felt as I came to terms with the enormity of my losses.

Being ill has cost me dearly. It has meant an end to my career aspirations, has limited my social life and forced a change of roles. Most of all I can no longer take it for granted that my body will function properly at any given time. I am having to deal with feelings of frustration, self-pity, despair and anger at the changes thrust upon me while at the same time learning to live with the inevitability of pain and discomfort. It is no wonder then that I sometimes envy others their uncomplicated lives.

What I needed most following diagnosis was for someone to mother me like I was still a child. I yearned for a mother's unconditional love, to be able to cry with my head on her lap, to draw strength from her once again. But as this was not available to me I had to go deep inside myself, learn to be my own beloved and make the strong decision to mother myself, for to heal I needed to take time for self-nurturing.

I had no choice but to slow down almost to the point of stopping altogether. This was difficult to accept and a struggle to achieve because my brain refused to slow down at the same pace as my body. It kept on working overtime long after my body had slowed right down. I was scared because I feared that once I allowed myself to stop I would not be able to start again.

Meeting the Challenge: Facing the Fear

I have progressed through cycles of mourning for the life I lost and sometimes fear stalks me, sapping my energy, power and will to go on. But I am learning to live beyond the fear by living through it and in the process learning to turn anger and frustration at my own limitations into creative energy. It is unlikely that I will be able to banish fear completely but I am learning to give it less space in my life and view it more as an occasional companion rather than waste energy fighting it. Learning to put fear into perspective has given me strength as well as recognition of the power I have within myself.

Although I feel that I have been very lucky in that there have been some gains from the very losses that I mourn, I wrestle with despair on a daily basis. An especially poignant time was when I succumbed to the flu virus again recently and went into relapse after a period of considerable progress. Acknowledging and accepting the vast impact ME has had on my life has consequently rendered the condition less important and is enabling me to move forward slowly. For example, last summer I was consumed with anger, very frightened, struggling to keep depression at bay and in a lot of pain. I had difficulty envisaging a future and when I did it appeared very bleak. In contrast I am now excited by the future and view the coming summer as a brand-new beginning, a welcome gift waiting to be opened, and wherever it leads me I willingly follow.

I have had to re-evaluate and re-organise my entire life. I am using this period to try and translate the pain and fear into strength, realising that I cannot wait until they disappear before I resume my life. It is important to me that something positive emerges out of the emotional and physical pain I am experiencing. This illness now helps shape my thoughts; the words I speak; the way I act; how I view the present and my vision of the future, as well as what I see as my purpose in life.

Meeting the Challenges: Facing the Humiliation of Not Working

Becoming ill precipitated a huge reduction in my financial situation. I realised too that I had to create a new identity for myself as I lost the status connected to being a professional. I had to adopt new labels and identities, for example, disabled; poor; benefit recipient and chronically ill.

I was humiliated by having to apply for state benefit and almost having to justify being ill. I felt I had stepped backwards. I had marketable skills and a desire to work but my body had failed me. It would have been harsh enough to be forced to stand still but to step backwards – my loss of income, dreams, aspirations, accommodation and identity was devastating!

Sometimes I cannot believe that I have changed so much

in a matter of only months. I reminisce at the way I used to dress for work – that well-groomed, smart woman in suits and business dresses with briefcase and accessories – was she really me?

Slowly I recognise that the losses are a reality that must be integrated into a new sense of self. The absence of employment, finance and change of identity are a recurrent sadness, but it no longer dominates my life.

I have always had a passion for good books, but now that I frequently experience difficulty reading I am developing a deeper appreciation of art, the theatre, music and poetry. In some of my loneliest and darkest moments these become my only companions and I am indebted to those who have produced them.

I constantly remind myself that I have a responsibility to build joy, laughter and fun into my life and that I don't have to be strong; I can choose to just be.

Facing the Challenge: Re-entering the Social World

My overwhelming fear is that I will vegetate and so I want to maintain, as far as possible, some of the skills, knowledge and experience I developed during my career. A limited amount of voluntary work (three hours each week) as a therapy provides me with some degree of mental stimulation. The interaction with others assists me in maintaining work-related skills while also enabling me to remove the focus from myself for short periods and thus helping to combat the depression which is always threatening to surface.

Outside of voluntary work, I have been able to build on old friendships. This period of illness has served as a real test of who my friends are. I have invested time and energy in friendships throughout my life and now the dividends are being returned to me with bonuses. Friends have rallied around offering encouragement and comfort. Initially I found it difficult to elicit support, even more so to accept it. Those friends who had supported me throughout the time I spent in Durham, had sustained the distance and absence maintaining contact primarily through letters and telephone calls. They kept in contact regardless of how long it took me to respond; and they are the ones who are still supporting me now that I am ill. Only now, a year after being diagnosed, am I able to accept their offers of visits and embrace fully the support they offer so unselfishly. I am now able to spend time with them and am just delighted that they persevered and refused to give up on me.

They are all different, complementing each other and offering strengths in different areas. Some concentrate on keeping me on track, reminding me of the journey we have travelled together; reassuring me that I will bounce back again; they encourage me to just allow myself the space to heal. Others assist me in maintaining my sense of humour while valuing and motivating me. It is reassuring to know that I am just as important to them now as I was prior to the illness. They demand nothing in return except my company and that I keep positive.

Meanwhile, my children are young adults and are returning to me a measure of what I gave to them when they were entirely dependent on me. We are seeing each other differently – I am becoming increasingly aware of their strengths and they are becoming accustomed to my vulnerability.

Conclusion

As the healing process begins I am appreciating the space to think and tap into my creativity, and relishing the opportunity to take control of my time and explore new challenges to replace those my career offered. Initially I resented the surplus time as I could do no more than observe others while they pursued their busy lives. I now welcome the freedom to plan and define my days, using them to engage in some of the activities I had always yearned to include in my life but lacked the space. For example, I have always acknowledged the importance of giving something back to society through voluntary work. Now it also serves as a reminder of how much I still have to offer in spite of being afflicted with a chronic illness. I still get frustrated periodically, and accept that this may remain so for some time yet, but I have moved steadily from denial of the illness to a place where I can now begin to accept it and appreciate that, although devastating, the experience of it is enriching my life in ways I never thought possible.

For the whole of my life, I have had to bend, sometimes with and at times against, the wind in order to survive this far. I am not about to give up now.

Lost

Aspen

I'm lost
in a sinking feeling
hollow
bereft,
my friends
have gone walking
and I remember what it's like

excited adventurers
    easy companionship
        eager feet,

memories crowd
leaving me
swamped.

I omitted
plans
slipped into
emptiness
without direction
but will not play
a losing game

a womanly trick
assuages such pain
and changes the view:
comforting music
a nice tablecloth
a date for one
with a good meal
and a book:

I hope they don't come home
before I do

Part Four

Benefits, Rights and Beyond

Benefits

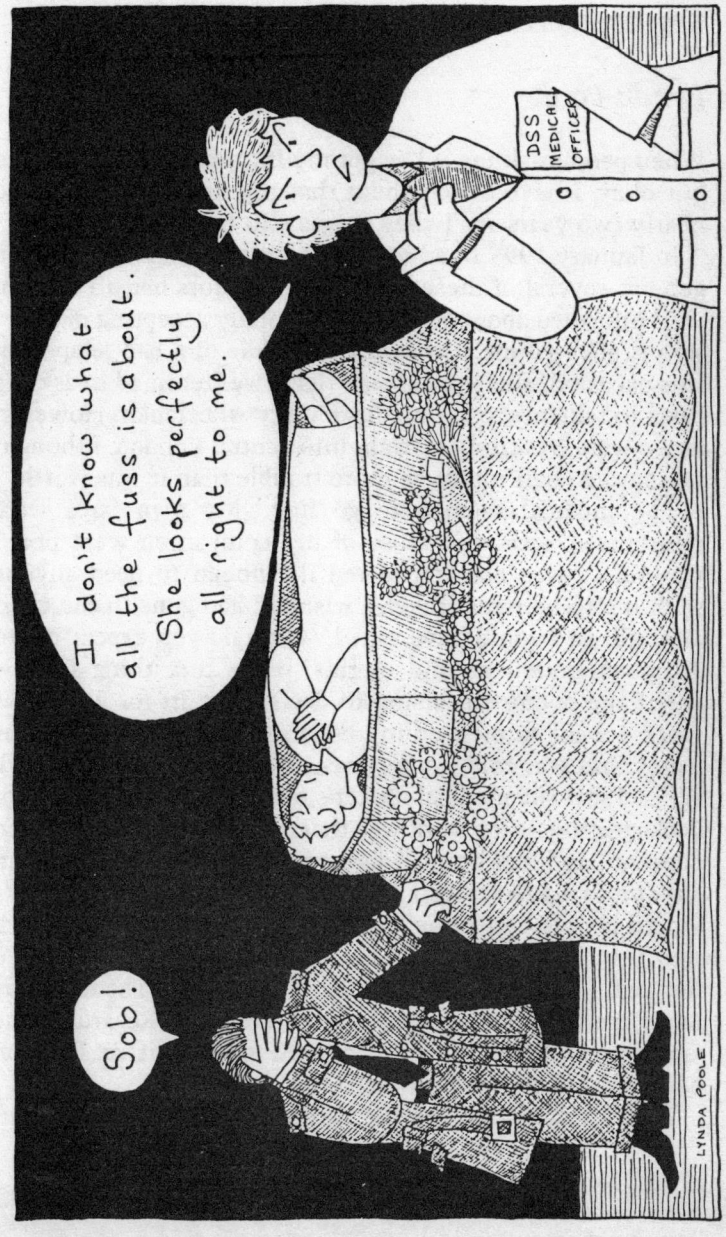

She Looks All Right to Me

Lynda Poole

When people ask me if I've got my Incapacity Benefit sorted out okay, I have to tell them that my money was stopped nearly two years ago (when it was still Invalidity Benefit).

In January 1995 I had to attend a routine DSS medical. I'd gone to several of these before – the doctors had all seemed well informed about ME, and were totally accepting of how I said it affected me. I was in the middle of a bad relapse on this occasion, and felt so weak that I was tempted to ask my carer to take me to the medical in my wheelchair. However, as we were travelling by train into central London, I thought taking the chair might be more trouble than it was worth.

The medical seemed to go fine. (My own fares were reimbursed, although those of my companion were not. I was told I was not considered ill enough to need anyone with me to help me travel. I wished I had gone in the chair after all, so I could have asked, 'What do you expect me to do, push myself around in this?') The first thing I knew about the doctor's decision to declare me fit for work was when I went to pick up my benefit from the post office as usual, and was told my payment book had been cancelled. When I saw the medical officer's report, the reason given for declaring me fit for work was that 'I looked well and seemed cheerful, and had been ill long enough.' I know better than anyone that I have been ill quite long enough, thank you. I would love to call 'time'. But unfortunately it doesn't work that way. I was surprised she could say I 'looked well' – I'd felt awful that day, and didn't expect a doctor to be fooled by any superficial appearances to the contrary. Regarding the 'seeming cheerful' bit, I do try hard to be positive. How on earth do you cope otherwise?

I appealed against the DSS medical officer's decision. But

the appeal went against me too. I was denied permission to present leaflets from the ME Association, outlining how the illness affects people in chronic cases. I was told everyone present 'already knew all about ME', and so didn't need to see this information. In the end, the opinion of the DSS medical officer, who had never seen me before, and only assessed me for about 15 minutes, was taken to outweigh my own testimony and the written evidence of my GP, consultant and carer.

Over a year later, I am still waiting for the last possible stage of my appeal to be heard. I cannot believe the amount of stress, emotional upset and financial hardship caused by one person basing their professional assessment of my health on how bright and cheerful I looked. Let's face it – doctors can still say ME is all in the mind. Even those who are more sympathetic hardly seem to be filled with a great sense of urgency to find a cure or effective treatment for the illness. Over six years ago, I was offered Interferon treatment by the consultant I was seeing at the time. I refused, wary of the potential side effects, especially as it had not been shown to be effective against ME. This year my new consultant offered me the chance to take part in an experimental programme looking into the same drug. It still hasn't been proven to work. On my most recent visit, he referred me to another researcher who needed volunteers. She explained how she wanted to monitor people over two days of treadmill tests 'done to the point of exhaustion'. (Yes, she said, some patients had relapsed afterwards, but 'not too severely'.) Her aim was to establish 'once and for all' whether people with ME 'really do' experience greater fatigue after exertion, or whether 'they just think they do'.

If I weren't trying so hard to stay positive, it really would start to get me down.

The Well of Creativity

Kate Cargreaves and Caeia March

December 1996

Dear Kate,

I have so enjoyed our exchange of letters since the start of this book project and have had in mind for ages to luxuriate in time out to reply. So here I am at last.

You asked me the technical stuff about therapeutic earnings: this is a tricky one depending on the vagaries of local GPs and local DSS but I have been lucky. I have also been businesslike and have taken advice from the Citizens' Advice Bureau. In any case the computers for Inland-Revenue and DSS are now compatible and linked so I feel it is always wise to take advice and play it by the rule book. Anything else is or can be classified as fraud. It's important to be up front and to be careful with this.

Firstly one declares all income annually to the Inland Revenue. My income would therefore be a) Incapacity Benefit, and b) writing as a separate and self-employed income.

Some writers don't declare bits and pieces of their money but none of us gets paid cash for writings – so it is all recorded somewhere, and therefore declarable.

If we are on Incapacity Benefit we have around forty pounds a week or thereabouts (check current level with CAB) 'disregard' before tax if we receive remuneration at any level. This is quite different from anyone on unemployment benefit or ordinary sickness benefit. It seems to me that it arises from a throwback to the iniquitous value system of the deserving and the undeserving poor that came from the 1834 Poor Law, which I studied in Sociology, years ago.

It seems to me that this value system is being reasserted, tightened horribly, to take as many of us back into the undeserving category as possible – off Incapacity Benefit and on to the dole. People on the dole can more easily be labelled negatively by all those in power – for it is said that they aren't searching hard enough to find jobs. If we are sick, then we are let off this negative judgement – it's argued that it's not our fault we're not at work, unless of course we are seen to be prolonging our sickness deliberately or not trying hard enough to get ourselves well and back to work. Then the system falls on us again.

This underlies the concept of therapeutic earnings: people on Incapacity Benefit are expected to do everything they can to get themselves well, off benefit and back to work. This concept of self-help to get back to work is complex around ME. Some people in official institutions – benefits, DSS doctors and so forth – really don't believe in ME. Neither do some consultant psychiatrists. Just try a bit harder, dear. It's all in the mind. Pull yourself together. Stop malingering – and all of that.

The fact remains that we are caught in a system that makes us keep proving we are ill, justifying ourselves, and begging for a pittance. It's stressful and wrong and none of this should be happening, however nice individual officials might be. Other women with ME have had awful experiences and have met up with horrible officials in different parts of the country.

So always start with the CAB, check out your rights carefully in the current economic climate and in the local situation. And always, no matter what, describe your symptoms on your worst day, as we have said, so many times.

Any activity that assists your ability to deal with and manage your symptoms, and helps you stay positive and potentially return to health can come under the umbrella of therapeutic earnings.

Money is never value free in this or any other society the world over. However, this 'disregard of earnings' does help us as women with a chronic illness – we can state validly, and without having to tell lies, that 'we need something to do to take our minds off our symptoms and to strengthen our confidence and encourage us to return to health'. That is more or less the official terminology. What it means is that we don't have to lie around or sit around all day staring at walls with no hope and no creativity. We are officially 'allowed' to have 'hobbies', i.e. things to do.

The all important issue is whether we are able to do full-time work of any kind. This is linked to the fitness for work test which we all dread. I am now classified as unable to work – which is true in terms of regular part-time/full-time gainful employment.

If on the other hand someone is on the dole, then to admit to writing would be complex – and difficulties would arise. Someone who writes, paints or plays music might be seen as making themselves unavailable for full-time work: it's dodgy and always best to seek advice.

As far as Incapacity Benefit goes – the procedure is that the DSS can suggest that you go to the doctor to get a letter about therapeutic earnings. The wording is important. It should say something along the lines I have suggested. Don't go alone to a GP who might not be aware or careful. Only go alone if you are confident that your GP will support you. If not, take a tough friend who stays with you and gives you the confidence to explain what you need in the letter.

The way I see it is that my creativity *is* my healing process. I not only have the right to be creative, whatever form it takes, but my mental and physical health depend on it. Personally this is so true for me, that I could assert it anywhere. But I still fear 'the system' because I understand its power and its values. I hate being on benefit but I have to have the money.

As it happens, the tax office smile gently at my annual statements because I make no profit from my writing though I am just over the threshold of breaking even. It pays for itself, and keeps me sane. Sometimes this low financial reward surprises people because of my output. But any author will say the same – many people who write make their living from teaching workshops, or giving public presentations of their work, not from royalties. The difference would be to have a film or television series or something. But such things are rare and do not apply to many novelists and poets.

But it's still an offence not to declare any income from writing either as a tax offence or as DSS fraud. Simply not worth it, I feel.

The DSS take a while to assess the GP's letter but there's nothing to lose. You only get to know it is accepted by default, i.e. if it wasn't, the benefit would stop. You don't have to do anything else re the DSS and they don't need to know how much you earn so long as it isn't over the amount of 'disregard'. But you'd have to be making two thousand a year profit from writing to take it over forty a week, so there's not much chance of that unless you get into films. Live in hope!

Kate, I'm ever so tired, suddenly. Going back to bed for an hour or so, will post this tomorrow and will write again soon.

Take care. Talk to you soon,
Love from Caeia xxx

7 May 1997

Dear Caeia,

It was so good to talk on the phone. I so enjoyed hearing bits about your life in Cornwall and know that when it's practical I really should move out of town and away to where the air has the same effect on my health. Meantime we just try to get away whenever we can – my sister has a caravan in West Wales and I love that area. There's a place in North Pembrokeshire called Abereiddy which gives me such a lift – I can actually walk the cliffs there, even if I do hobble for days afterwards!

I'm sorry for the delay, but here's the information re Severe Disablement Allowance and therapeutic earnings. Basically it's the same as with Incapacity Benefit. With your doctor's backing and DSS approval you can work for up to 16 hours per week and earn up to £46.50 per week (that's from April '97) while claiming either Incapacity Benefit or SDA.

The £46.50 is after you deduct 'certain expenses' e.g. fares to work, union subs etc. I don't know whether costs of writing – ink cartridges/ribbons, postage, phone calls etc. count as 'certain expenses'. A DSS fact sheet says the work must clearly be seen as 'beneficial' to recovery or as 'therapy'.

As for the Disability Living Allowance which we discussed on the phone, I've been on the mobility component for a few years now. DLA has two components – mobility and personal care but I only need the former. To qualify for that, you have to be able to prove that you are seriously restricted in mobility, and to get the personal care component, that you need assistance to care for yourself. It would take some time to detail how it's all worked out, but anyone who is unable to walk easily because of ME and/or needs someone to look after them, cook meals for them, etc., should call the Benefits Enquiry Line on freephone 0800 882200. I've been able to get the benefit on the basis that walking causes me severe discomfort and makes all my symptoms much worse. I look perfectly okay when walking a short way, incidentally, so people shouldn't be put off applying if they don't use a wheelchair or walking stick, etc. (although I now use a scooter, I didn't when I first received DLA). A friend has the personal care on top of the mobility because her ME is bad enough for her to need her family to prepare her meals, wash her hair, etc.

However, applicants need to be wised up to how the system works. It's crucial, as you say, always to talk in terms of how you are *at your worst*, not what you can do on better days. I had a nasty shock two years ago when my application for DLA renewal was turned down arbitrarily, even though I was no better. I applied for a review of the decision and set about proving my entitlement like a military campaign. Someone I know had her application for renewal turned down just before Christmas one year. She had it granted on review, but her Christmas was ruined and she had to wait five months for the review. Her health was made much worse with the stress of it all too. So I was determined to get it sorted out as quickly as possible.

The Benefit Enquiry Line advised me to get strong medical backing and the Benefits Adviser of Action for ME told me that I was entitled to an explanation for the rejection and to see all papers relating to my case. She also told me to focus my case entirely on *what happens to my body when I walk, and the collapse caused by over-exertion.*

I spent days writing letters and making phone calls. My MP and a doctor I had seen privately supported my claim and I have no doubt that helped me get the decision overturned within five weeks – though I hassled the DLA staff endlessly during that time too! I made it clear that I was writing to them and ringing them from my bed – it was a great strain as my SDA was dependent on my receiving the DLA, so I stood to lose both benefits.

I've just applied for the renewal of my DLA again and have sent copies of all the correspondence from that review and made it clear that I wouldn't take kindly to being put through it all again! Anyone applying for the first time, or fighting a similar rejection, should go through every little bit of information they give on their forms with a tooth comb – get a local authority Welfare Rights Officer to check it through or contact the CAB. The ME organisations have benefits advisors too. It's absolutely vital that doctors know the way the system works – my GP, who's very understanding, made the mistake of saying that 'on a good day she can be quite active' and I'm sure that did for me when the DLA renewal was initially refused. Being active is relative – my 'quite active' is a fit person's idea of a nightmare!

You can never really take it all for granted, as you've said – there's always the feeling that it could all be ended on the whim of an Adjudications Officer or a tightening of the criteria. I too dread the prospect of medicals etc. – I've only had one DSS medical, but that was enough. The doctor was brusque beyond belief, but to my intense relief he decreed that I was indeed unfit for work.

I absolutely agree that our creativity is our healing process. Without my writing I don't know how I would survive, and although I remain physically ill the writing has been profoundly healing in every other way. Even the weekly letter to a friend, however mundane, is part of it – sometimes it's all I can manage. And writing to/hearing from you is a joy.

All for now and take care – enjoy the garden! The spring bulbs must be wonderful.

Love, Kate xxx

All Work and No Pay: Campaigning to Scrap the Incapacity Act

Kate Adams

In June 1994 the Incapacity for Work Act, a piece of legislation which would have serious consequences for disabled people, passed through Parliament, virtually unnoticed.

Under the new law, Sickness and Invalidity Benefit, the main income of thousands of people unable to work because of poor health and impairments, was renamed Incapacity Benefit. Benefit rates and allowances were cut and a new draconian 'All Work Test' was introduced, deciding eligibility. The new benefit assessment no longer looked at whether you could do a job, given the constraints of ill health, or at the possibility of available work that was also accessible. It simply and crudely measured a set of physical and mental functions. So if someone could pick up a bag of potatoes or a pint of milk or could read a magazine and answer the telephone, it would count against them. They would lose points at their DSS examination and might subsequently lose their benefit.

The only publicity that accompanied this iniquitous change to a crucial part of the welfare state system was an announcement by Social Security Minister Peter Lilley that he intended to clamp down on benefit fraud. Half a million long-term sick and disabled people would be removed from benefit over three years, saving the country £1.5 billion. The money would now only go to 'genuine claimants'.

Lilley had no evidence to back this smear. He relied on existing prejudice and discrimination. Ironically the Disabled People's Civil Rights Campaign, centred at the time on MP Roger Berry's Private Member's Bill, provided a distraction rather than a challenge to the social security legislation. The Conservative Government, by sneaking the Incapacity Bill through Parliament when attention was focused elsewhere, exercised clever timing. Shots of campaigners in wheelchairs blocking buses, which were shown on TV, presented a view of disability that was based on obvious physical impairment. People with invisible and fluctuating conditions like asthma, RSI, HIV, Mental Health and, of course, ME were not represented in the media coverage. The threat to their income by the Incapacity for Work Act, and the effect this would have on their health and their lives, was not reported either. This indirectly reinforced Peter Lilley's false distinction between genuine and fraudulent claimants.

When I found out about the proposed benefit changes I was horrified and telephoned various disability organisations, including the Disabled Members' section of my trade union, hoping to discover some resistance. Most people didn't know what I was talking about. Charities said they could not take political action. Activists were preoccupied with the civil rights struggle; they did not see income rights for disabled people as part of that political agenda. Eventually I realised that the real opposition would have to come from claimants themselves.

I met up with three other people with ME who were prepared to do something and one person who had experience in direct-action protests around HIV and AIDS. We were assisted with information from the organisation The Disability Alliance and practical support from my non disabled partner. We decided to call a protest outside Peter Lilley's Islington town house. Forty people attended the demonstration. We had a march, shouted loudly and stopped the traffic on a zebra crossing. It was a lot of fun, nerve-racking and quite exhausting. Incapacity Action, the campaign to repeal the Incapacity for Work Act, was born.

Two years and several demonstrations later, Incapacity Action is still up and running. We have no proper funding or office resources and exist on donations, working from home. We keep going because we are angry and want justice for ourselves and all disabled claimants. The Incapacity for Work Act has taken millions of pounds from disabled people and brought untold stress and pressure into their lives. It has to go.

Many of the original campaigners in Incapacity Action have dropped out because of the strain on their health, but new people have joined with fresh ideas and inspiration. For myself, the best part has been a connection with other disabled people, fighting for something really important. I have severe ME and sometimes the responsibility and the effort involved has felt too much. Equally it has been far better to do this than to stay silent.

Disability and Rights

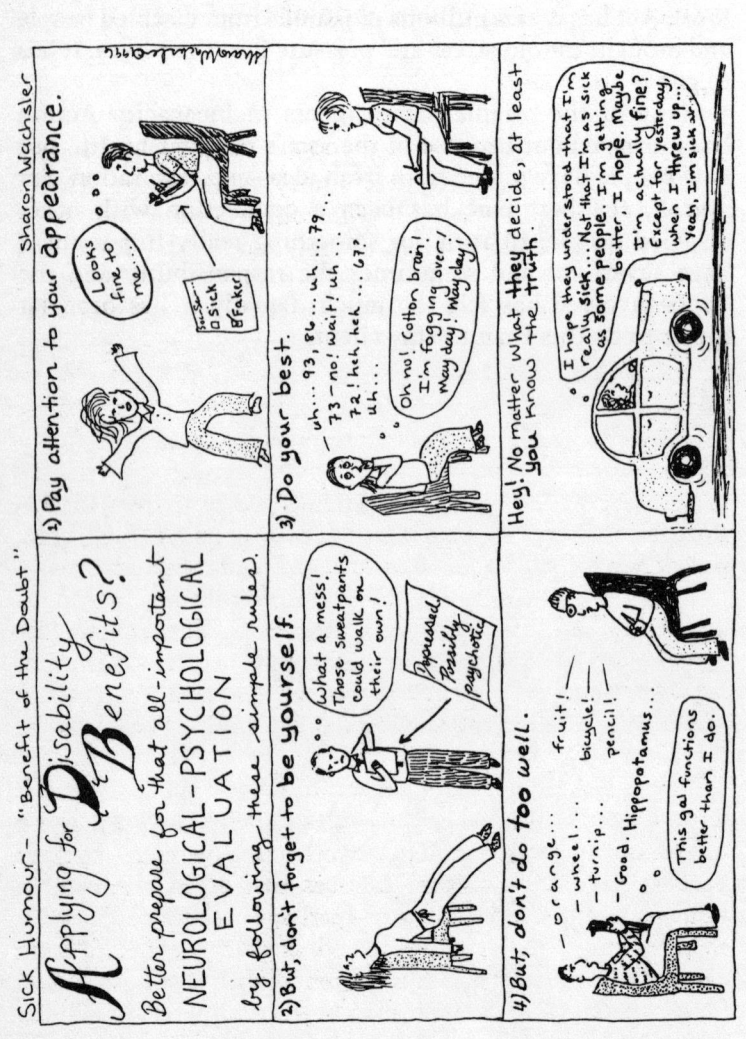

Staggering to the Other Side of the Fence

Sharon Wachsler

From 1991 through most of 1995, I was an able-bodied member of the disability community. After having studied the disability rights movement in college, I went on to work in the field of disability information and referral. Disability issues pervaded every aspect of my life: I sent letters to politicians advocating housing rights for people with disabilities; I became friends with people with epilepsy, fibromyalgia, Chronic Fatigue Immune Dysfunction Syndrome (CFIDS), and deafness; I watched as my close (previously healthy) friend developed CFIDS and Multiple Chemical Sensitivity (MCS); and every month at work I'd take hundreds of phone calls from people with every kind of disability, trying to help them locate housing, food, jobs, personal care assistance, financial aid, and other services.

In my work, where so many callers told me of sudden accidents and life-changing illnesses, I was continually confronted by how random and fragile the distinction is between being able-bodied and being disabled. Particularly when they were young and female, I'd think, 'This could be me.'

I had an especially strong reaction when I spoke to people with CFIDS, fibromyalgia, or MCS. Perhaps because these disorders disproportionately affect young women; perhaps because they are systemic diseases that affect a person in numerous and mysterious ways; perhaps because people with these disorders tend to be treated as crazy or 'fakers'; and certainly because I had close friends with CFIDS, MCS, and fibromyalgia, I took an increasingly greater interest in helping callers with these disabilities. Often, after such a call, I would think, 'My God, I hope this never happens to *me*.'

These thoughts were far from my mind in the fall of 1995.

Overworked and happy, I was teaching self-defence classes, biking every day to my full-time job, swimming and pursuing my dream career in sign language interpreting.

It was at this time, however, that I began getting sick frequently. Initially for a few days at a time and then for weeks at a stretch I would become dizzy, nauseated, headachy, incredibly tired, and tormented by a bizarre feeling of unreality. I spent every day lying on the couch, often too sick even to read or watch television. Doctors found nothing to explain my symptoms and suggested psychiatric evaluations.

When I became sick in mid-October, I did not recover after a couple of weeks, as I had previously. Every week I'd tell my boss I might return 'next week'. Yet, as the weeks passed, my symptoms worsened and increased. I became painfully aware that what I was experiencing – low fever, sore throat, insomnia and cognitive impairments (such as memory loss and trouble concentrating) – were symptoms associated with CFIDS. I was in a panic, praying to be diagnosed with a disease that could be cured – anything but CFIDS. To my dismay, however, lab tests for other illnesses kept returning negative. Finally, in early December I saw a doctor who diagnosed me with CFIDS. I was so tired and out of it that at first I was numb, but as the news cut through my mental fog I was filled with despair. That night I called one friend after another and cried and cried.

By the next day, I felt only relief. I had been in a state of anxiety for so long, fearing the worst. Now that the worst had happened, I had nothing left to fear. Or so I thought. I set about adjusting to my new circumstances, gathering information, informing my friends and family, and trying to think positively about a new life with chronic illness.

One of the scariest aspects of CFIDS is that it makes one highly susceptible to MCS. But because I had never before had allergies, I thought it unlikely that I would develop chemical sensitivities. I was wrong. Two days after my diagnosis I was lying in bed while a helper mopped the floors. The smell of the floor cleaner rose in a wave, overwhelming me. I suddenly got very 'spacy' and dizzy. My eyes itched, and I began to wheeze and cough. Desperate to get relief, I staggered around the apartment, opening all the windows. Later that day a co-worker visited me. He was wearing cologne, and again I was knocked flat by asthma and mental confusion. I knew from the power and immediate nature of my responses that I had developed chemical sensitivities. I was devastated.

Everybody who becomes disabled has reactions of grief, denial, fear and anger. I am no exception. However, I think my unique situation of having been in the disability community before I got sick has made some of the process different for me.

For one thing, I think that I knew I had CFIDS and started to accept it as a life-changing illness much faster than most. The other women I know who have CFIDS tried for months or even years to attend work or school, even though it was making them very sick. Because I recognised my symptoms as being similar to my friends', I knew my condition was serious and did not attempt to 'push through' the illness. Furthermore, acceptance and successful coping are much easier when one's supporters are not ignorant of the disease or in denial about it. I've heard other women with CFIDS speak about trying to hide their illness from their friends, or struggling to make them understand why going out all the time and partying is no longer possible. Since all my close friends have physical limitations, I can bask in frequent empathetic telephone conversations. I get affirmation about what I'm experiencing physically, mentally and emotionally. The one drawback to relying on other sick people is that it is extra difficult for them to get out of the house to visit or provide assistance.

I must admit that I do feel an odd mixture of acceptance and disbelief about having become sick with the very illness to which I had devoted such passion and energy when I was able-bodied. On the one hand, my work in the disability community has led me to see disability as a part of life –

something that can affect anyone. In that respect it seems perfectly natural and unsurprising that I got sick. On the other hand, it feels bizarrely coincidental and ironic that I am educating my family and distant friends about my condition by giving them copies of the same fact sheets that I wrote at work when I was healthy. From a practical standpoint this prior knowledge has really paid off: I've known where to go for information on treatments, a good doctor, and a support group. Likewise, when I've had to apply for disability-related services and benefits, I've relied on the advice I used to give to others.

In addition to helping with the 'where' and 'how' parts of a new disability, my background has laid the 'why' questions to rest. It's a natural human response to a crisis to ask 'Why me? Why now? What have I done to deserve this?' I did a little bit of that, I admit. But for the most part, those questions were answered for me long before I got sick. I've spoken with enough people with disabilities to know that it can and does happen to anyone. In addition, people I love and respect have disabilities. It never occurred to me to blame them. In this way I have been able to let myself off the hook also.

By the same token, after years of using the 'correct' vocabulary about disability, the respect and dignity it conveys has entered my soul and now helps to cushion me against those who don't understand and against my own self-doubts. In a society where women 'should' be self-sufficient (working), active (athletic), and beautiful (able-bodied, at least), I have been lucky to experience remarkably little shame in being disabled. I have new insight into the dehumanisation of words like 'pity', 'tragedy', and 'courageous', I know that those words do not apply to me.

Another powerful word often used in the context of disability is 'inspiring'. Despite its potentially derogatory connotations, as in reference to the 'inspiring true story of the crippled girl who beat the odds', I have truly found inspiration from other women with disabilities. As I try to adapt to a new life that requires a new identity, my friends with disabilities have provided me with excellent role models. From one, I can learn hope and perseverance for recovery; from another, acceptance and pride in a life fully lived despite sickness. From those who work, I understand about asking for accommodations and juggling conflicting needs; from those who don't, I learn that there are ways that I can give back to the community and to myself without doing paid work. Considering how hidden the real lives of women with disabilities are, I'm grateful for the abundance of true 'success stories' around me.

It's hard to conclude a story that's at its beginning in so many ways. Despite my supports, it's a struggle to be newly sick, and with every new challenge I take on, I discover several limitations. I'm still adjusting, still discovering and mourning new losses. I miss the life I had before CFIDS and MCS destroyed it. But if I had to get sick, I'm grateful that it was after having become a part of the disability community. I joke with my friends with CFIDS that I'm standing on the shoulders of those who got sick before me, and that's probably why they're so tired all the time.

In the Open

Amanda Cornu

Part of the human race,
People sit and stare,
I watch and contemplate
No longer housebound
In a lonely bed.
With rays of sunshine
streaming through
On a platform
a black drummer
performs, exudes life.
The sound of drums
Resounding, reminders of life
I feel myself uncurl
Cry, scream out
my very soul on fire
With a lust for life
A desire to live.
While I remember
My invalid bed awaits
Hours alone, bereft
Boredom and Inaction, Abounding.

ME and Disability

Julia Cameron

Ours is a devilish illness to manage, with its unpredictability and fluctuations, and we have all searched for ways of coping with what is happening to us. We have not just needed strategies to cope physically; ways of making sense of our altered lives, of creating meaningfulness out of our disarray, have been just as vital. For me, one such strategy has been to consider myself a disabled person.

I admit this viewpoint may not appeal to everyone; in fact it may terrify some people, and it may not be appropriate or helpful for those who have not had ME long. But I have had a form of chronic fatigue for over 20 years, although I spent most of that time hiding my lack of resilience even from myself. I worked part-time for many years and kidded myself this was a choice. I danced, swam, cycled and generally gave an impression of activity and zest. Because I worked part-time I was able to do these things *and* keep my immune system more or less functional. I still got more bugs than most people, but I was able to be secretive about the frequency of my infections since I did not work five days a week. Thus I kept my jobs and a charade of fitness.

Fitness, as we who lack it know only too well, is highly prized in our culture. To be without it is to be lesser in some way, 'in-valid', of reduced worth and importance, morally and psychically weak, damaged goods. Having had, like most of us, such oppressive messages spoon-fed from childhood, it is no wonder I hid my sickness even from myself.

My strategy for survival worked more or less for a long time. But in 1989, during that phase when a particularly virulent strain of Coxsackie was on the rampage throughout the world, I became suddenly and acutely ill. My damaged immunity, which had struggled so womanfully to cope since being attacked repeatedly by Septrin many years before, succumbed almost completely to this viral assault. I could no longer con myself I was 'fit'; I could no longer 'pass' as one of them, the well people.

As acute illness was superseded by the classic brain and muscle symptoms of ME, one of the multitude of emotions and reactions I had was relief at dropping the pretence that I was a member of that other species. I was so obviously ill, unfit, that deceit had to be fully dispensed with. It was only a short stop from that to recognising my identity as a disabled person.

Since coming out as disabled I have started to learn about and gain great encouragement from the 'social model' of disability. This theory was developed by disabled activists to challenge the discrimination and segregation which still flows from the ethos of the 'medical model' of disability.

The medical model equates 'disability' with 'impairment'. It says you are disabled by what is 'wrong' with you. This has many implications, one of which is the creation of divisions and lack of understanding between disabled people themselves, as well as between the disabled and the non-disabled. We can see this very clearly in the role of charities which 'help' disabled people with differing impairments, going 'cap in hand' to the public and playing on the image of disabled people as tragic beings who need pity and handouts.

The social model looks at impairment quite differently, seeing it as totally distinct from disability, which is the way you are discriminated against or excluded from participation in society. With the social model it is society, not some individual bodily dysfunction, which creates disability. For example, lack of wheelchair access to most buildings and almost all public transport disables people who cannot walk; their leg impairment is not the disabling issue, the way the physical environment is constructed is. Similarly, the fact that very few people know British Sign Language disables those deaf people who rely on it for communication. It is not their lack of hearing which is making them 'not able', but attitudes, education and society's expectations.

With ME the picture is more complex. There are some conditions and impairments for which if 'disability' were removed, 'impairment' would cease to be a problem, but there are conditions where even if society was completely fair and non-discriminatory we would still on balance choose not to have the impairment. Conditions that are life-threatening come into this category, and arguably so does ME, quality-of-life threatener par excellence.

But the social model is just as relevant to us as to someone with a more straightforward impairment where continued dysfunction is a certainty. I have found it a positive and strengthening exercise to think what my life would be like if I only had the impairment of ME and none of the disability which at present is its inevitable companion.

What would it be like if we never again had to contend with offensive media items about 'yuppie flu' or suggestions from parts of the medical profession that this was a form of hysteria? What would it be like if the disruption and devastation which ME can cause were fully recognised and adequate funds were pumped into research into immunology, virology and cellular functioning? What if people with the illness were really taken seriously, so that incidents like those of children being thrown into hydrotherapy pools because their word and that of their parents was not believed were seen as the cruel torture of an unenlightened, bygone era?

What would it be like if the benefits and employment systems were flexible enough to enable us to slowly reintegrate into work as and when we began again to have the energy, without fear of losing money? Where anyone who needed more than a minuscule amount of sick leave was not fired immediately? Where a several-year gap between jobs on your application form or CV did not mean it was automatically binned? Where work was available in varied time segments, so that a job with a living wage did not mean at least 36 hours, week in week out?

What would it be like if in addition to automatic wheel-chair access there were comfortable chairs with headrests at cinemas, theatres, meeting venues? If there were 'rest areas' with quiet places to lie down at stations, shopping centres or workplaces? If there were widespread community facilities to help with the care of children and adult dependants? And what would it be like if the world were not driven along at ever greater speed by technological and business interests at the pace of the fastest and fittest, leaving behind those increasing numbers who cannot keep up?

Part of the impairment of ME is undoubtedly caused by the way society disables those of us who have it. A more relaxed pace of life; less stress induced by worries about jobs, benefits and resulting poverty; really adequate care services; and rest areas in public places, for example, would improve a lot of our symptoms and enable us to participate more fully in the world. As well as making life healthier and more enjoyable for everyone else . . .

It could be argued that acknowledging my disabled identity simply mires me in illness, that it denies the possibility of recovery and renewal. But the truth is that even if my impairment disappears tomorrow I will still be disabled: I have not worked for seven years, and because of that my chances in the job market will be very unequal. I may recover, I aim to do so, but disability will still affect me.

As it is I have a vision, developing all the time, of how the world could be, a vision which gives me joy and lessens my feelings of isolation, frustration and gloom. A vision which reminds me how well I am doing rather than what a wretched failure I am, which helps me take pride in having survived with an impairment which is still widely treated with disbelief and contempt. And which gives me a sense of common purpose with the many other people who are thinking about and working towards such a vision; it means I think of myself as part of a civil rights movement fighting for social change which will ultimately benefit everyone.

This strengthens me against the isolation which is such a key facet of life with ME. With this attitude I remind myself that my exclusion is not an inevitable part of the illness, but a result of current social construction, and thus open to challenge.

Smile Sandwich

Aspen

An Outside Smile

'God loves you.'

A hot voice has licked my forehead. I am stopped. I turn. I am confronted by a sweating face.

She looks confused as she searches for something relevant to say. Her hand is squeezing my arm. Her mouth opens into a smile so big I am falling between her teeth. She crunches my face, eats me, digests me and makes me part of the reality she understands. I am blemished in her eyes. I must have sinned. She pities me.

'God loves you.' She drops two leaflets into my lap. They invite me to attend her church.

I feel emotionally assaulted. I am gnashing and spitting and bored all at once. She has thrust herself into my life without invitation. She is wasting my time. Her attitude to me is showing in her smile, like a big turd on her face. It's her shit. I don't want it sticking to me.

Inside Smiles

Waves of welcome roll over me as I enter the writing workshop for disabled women.

Someone cracks a joke about my sun-lounger. The laughter splashes like seaspray. I test the water. It's warm. Smiles offer me big towels and a bag of chips after my swim. I wade in.

Outside Smiles

'I used to wear one of those,' the woman says, pointing to my neck collar. I am not remotely interested.

'Did you have an accident?' she asks, looking at my wheelchair.

I turn to ask my lover to push me on.

'Did someone do that to you?' the woman persists. Her hand slithers down my arm. My nerves shrink. I feel polluted. Her mouth trembles at the edge and I am covered in syrup.

'Please push me on.' Not polite. Angry.

My lover's daughter is shocked. She smiles apologetically at the 'understanding' woman.

I feel an eruption of lava which coagulates at the gates, gagging me.

The woman was only being friendly and sympathetic, daughter explains. She smiles as if I am a hopeless case, impossible, so touchy, so embarrassing.

When I get my electric wheelchair I will leave nosy members of the public standing.

Rebuke

Meg Torwl

in-valid
victim
sufferer
bedridden
wheelchair bound
pull your own weight
stand alone
stand on your own
two feet
four feet .
six legs
six feet under
dig your toes in
keep a lid on it
under your hat
sit on it
sit tight
don't just sit there
rise above it
get up
stand up for your rights
relax
take it easy
footloose
one foot in front t'other
one step at a time
walk before you can run
look before you leap
for the high jump
take: a running jump
a flying leap

a hike
put your foot in it
can't stand it
don't take it lying down
sleep on it
put it behind you
move on
walk away
turn away
turn the other cheek
a nod's as good as a wink
tunnel vision
blind
dumb
deaf
get a grip
hold on
handle it
give me a hand
can't stomach it
made my stomach turn
gutless
lily-livered
got a gall
spineless
heartless
thoughtless
some nerve
brain dead
uncommunicative
non-responsive
life sucked out
coming up for air
gasping
give me some air
breathing space
stood in good stead
stood me up

just stood by
gawking
dribbling on
stand firm
stand tall
stand and deliver
money or your life

Muscle Fetish

Aspen

A dyke said to me,
'don't you love it when those
      tasty women athletes
all pumping blood and oxygen
power through
some personal hurdle?'

I love it
when my friend asks me to comb her hair
so her strength is free to paint
intricate visions just for herself.

I love it
when she sings
taking minute gasps of air between
each tiny sound, cascades of melody
so light they're almost gone
before they reach my ears.

I love it when her worn-out, pressured
muscles, trembling with the onslaught
of a workout she never chose, the burn
which seldom stops, feel a hiatus
which allows her to move and dance.

Dykes dribble over the muscles of dykes
   who walk the hills
   who mend cars
   who dance till dawn
but ignore dykes
   who lie all day in bed
   who cannot direct their muscles
   whose muscles tire easily.

Patriarchy told us we mustn't have muscles
but when they bowl we don't have to bat . . .
we can refuse to play cricket.

You lust after muscles
I lust for spirit.
Watch out for the spirit of disabled dykes
you may not be able to take
such strength.

When is a Disability Not a Disability?
When It's ME

Anna Ravetz

The first summer I was ill, my body's capabilities changed rapidly. I could not stand up for more than a minute, and walks which I had previously not thought about – because they were so short – became literally unthinkable because I could not do them. I felt extremely ill, and exhausted, all the time.

The effect on me was profound. Among other things, I felt extremely embarrassed because I was not 'normal'. I felt that I was upsetting to other people, and that this made me a bad person. I had an agonising feeling that my actions must seem very strange. I wanted to explain why I was hardly walking, why I hardly left my flat, why I could not pop down to see a neighbour, but I did not know how to. No one asked questions which would have given me an opening, and saying I had ME seemed of little use, because most people either had an imperfect understanding of ME, or had never heard of it.

After about a year, I began to wonder if, while I had ME, I was disabled. I did not believe I really had a right to use this label – in common with most people I had very hazy ideas about disability. I probably assumed that the word disabled referred to people who were 'confined' to wheelchairs for life. I could walk, I did not use a wheelchair, and I did not know how long I would be ill. Nor had anyone said to me I was disabled. Yet I hardly went out of the house, and one of the reasons was that I could only walk a few steps outside. I wondered if in some second-class way I might be disabled, and I found it a helpful label to use when I had to get a minicab – a short way of saying I would be slow answering the door.

Although I began to call myself disabled, I would not use a wheelchair – even though the distance I could walk was heartbreakingly short, and this severely limited what I could do. Like most people, I thought that people in wheelchairs were completely dependent and helpless. I thought that if I was seen in a wheelchair I would somehow become less of a person. Having lost so much already, I couldn't bear this and I certainly was not alone in my feelings in the ME world – as one reader wrote in the newsletter of the ME Association, 'The main reason for this letter is – please ME magazine, no more stories, articles, etc about *wheelchairs*.'[1]

But one day, I did use a wheelchair, because the situation, and the person I was with, were so persuasive. We were at a centre for gardening and I longed to see the gardens, but walking round was out of the question. But there was a wheelchair available, and my partner suggested we use it. Very reluctantly, I agreed; my biggest fear, that someone I knew would *see* me, did not seem likely to be realised as we were not near home.

As soon as I got into the chair, I experienced the strongest feeling of liberation I have ever felt in my life. To move around is both pleasurable and empowering; if your mobility is restricted, that is deprivation. I still feel that liberation every time I use a wheelchair.

That day I also scotched once and for all my own myth that there was 'no point' using a wheelchair because I felt so exhausted I could not go anywhere anyway. I discovered that preserving my physical energy, by not walking at all, had a very positive effect on my mental state: I felt a little less ill, less exhausted. This has been a most useful piece of knowledge in living with ME.

Soon after, I got a manual wheelchair from the NHS. Later, I bought an electric chair second-hand (I never liked being pushed). They have been very good for me. But I still have a complicated mixture of feelings about using them, of which more later.

Two years on, I met Vanessa. She was full of confidence and I was very attracted to her. She was the first person I had ever met who identified herself as disabled, and she had an understanding of disability which was new to me. She thought that disabled people had a very raw deal, but she questioned the reasons for this. Up till that point I had thought that disability was created by the things that didn't work in people's bodies. Vanessa thought that disability is created by the way society is organised. This was my first introduction to the 'social model' of disability.

The social model of disability is a way of conceptualising disability: what disability is, and what causes it. The ideas of the social model began developing in Europe and the USA in the 1970s.[2] Before the social model was developed, disability was understood to arise out of the impairments in a person's body: something missing or something not working. If these impairments meant that the person could not do something that an able-bodied person could do, she or he was disabled. The cause of the disability was the failure of his or her body to function. Many people still have this view of disability; it is sometimes known as the 'medical model' of disability.

The social model agrees that disabled people have impairments in their bodies. But why, it asks, do these impairments matter? The social model says that it matters because the world is designed for able-bodied people and takes very little account of people with impairments. Because of this, people with various kinds of impairments are automatically excluded from many different places and activities. It is this *exclusion* which creates disabilities, not the impairments. If the world were designed differently, so that it took account of all the different impairments, people with impairments would not be excluded, and so they would not be disabled.

The social model was an immensely important shift in consciousness. Before it emerged, the foundation of all ideas about disabled people was that there was something wrong with them because in some way they deviated from the normal. With the social model, the focus shifted. Now, the thing that was wrong was society, for failing to adapt to all the people in it. This meant that disabled people could begin to identify themselves as members of an oppressed group whose civil rights were being denied. They began to argue that their needs should be catered for within the mainstream: in areas such as transport, housing and education. Previous provision, if any, for disabled people had been segregated, and inferior. With the emergence of a number of campaigns and groups organised by disabled people, for themselves, it became possible to talk about the disability movement.

Vanessa died, suddenly and tragically, when I had just begun to know her. But I am certain that her influence will stay with me for the rest of my life.

After she died, I began to read about disability politics and to have some contact with the disability movement. Feminism had previously been a big influence on me, and it was disheartening to find how severely feminism had neglected disability issues.

I didn't feel completely at home in the disability movement. I continued to find it difficult to define myself. Sometimes, my contact with the movement amplified my earlier feeling that I was not 'really' disabled. Once, I had my knuckles rapped by a disabled activist. Claiming common ground with her, I was told rather sternly that there is a difference between illness and disability. There was a clear implication that she did not consider that I was disabled. I felt quite put down by this. Was it not the case that some illnesses could give you disabilities? But who am I to say, I thought – she is an activist, she must know . . . (I now believe that you can be both ill and disabled, although you can also be ill without being disabled, or vice versa).

I found that there were many differences between myself, disabled by illness in adulthood, and many of the people I met in the disability movement. People who were disabled from birth or from childhood had had experiences that I never had as an able-bodied child, and they experienced a level of oppression that I never will encounter. This made me question whether I really belonged in the disability movement at all – bringing me back to my old question of whether I was fraudulent to call myself disabled. But if I did accept that I was disabled, there seemed to be gaps in what parts of my experience I could share. It did not seem to be the done thing to talk about pain or exhaustion and how much this limited my life, and when I looked for understanding of my illness and its effect on me, I was as disappointed as when I sought understanding from the severely able-bodied. I am very glad that five years on from these early encounters I am starting to find writing that looks at the effects of different impairments on the people who have them, and the reasons why it has been difficult to talk about them.[3]

I hate to say it, but another of my problems with the disability movement is the social model of disability! I cannot say all my disabilities could be removed if society were different. Certainly, accessible buses would enable me to go further than the local shops in my wheelchair, when I feel too unwell to drive. Accessible buildings would put an end to those exhausting and infuriating times I have to bang on the door of the (supposedly staffed) back entrance for 'Goods and Disabled'. But I cannot think of any alteration in society which would change how I *feel* – the exhaustion, pain and malaise which so severely limit my energy. And it is the lack of energy which limits my life, as much as external barriers. If the world were totally accessible to wheelchairs, and social attitudes were completely tolerant, I would still have to spend a lot of my time resting at home. So the social model of disability does not completely address my experience. I am certainly not arguing that the social model is wrong. However, I have been interested to read work by a visually impaired woman, who would count as disabled by any reckoning, and who also believes that some of her problems are not amenable to social solutions.[4] One of the examples she gives is her inability to recognise people in the street. When she moved house, she explained this to her new neighbours, and they undertook to greet her when their paths crossed. Initially, they did so, but gradually the greetings tailed off. She feels that the encounters were strained because of her lack of recognition, and not rewarding enough for the neighbours to continue. She was trying to find a social solution to a problem arising out of her impairment, but it did not work, and this made her question whether the problem could be regarded as entirely socially created.

Nevertheless, I have gained a great deal from my contact with the disabled movement. I am much happier to use a wheelchair because my image of wheelchairs is now very positive. Maximising my energy, rather than desperately trying to appear able-bodied, is the most important thing in my life now, and I will use a wheelchair, and any other aids, if they help me to do this.

I still have uncomfortable feelings about using a wheelchair, but these are not related to the wheelchair itself, but to my intermittent use of it and what other people make of this. I fear that most people think that if you use a wheelchair at all, you use it all the time (the expression 'confined' to a wheelchair says it all). Wheelchairs are still seen as a total replacement for legs, not an alternative means of transport. But for me, it's quite normal to use it for shopping one day – but get out of it to go into an inaccessible shop – and the next, do errands locally on foot from my car (blessing the orange badge). *I* know the logic of all this but do other people understand? Or do they think that I am mad – or that the problems I speak of are all in my head ('I saw you walking up that road only yesterday!') – a dangerous position for any ME sufferer! What do my neighbours think when they see me strolling in and out of my house, apparently perfectly normally, then unloading my wheelchair from my car? What does it matter what they think? In one sense, nothing. But I feel that I am a different social being when I am in my wheelchair, and I dread confronting the confusion of people who see one social being – the wheelchair-using Anna – one minute, and another – the ambulant Anna – the next. The result is that I consciously avoid going to places in my wheelchair where people have been used to seeing me walking, and vice versa. I must say, however, in fairness to my friends, acquaintances and neighbours, I have never heard a comment which casts doubt on my need for the wheelchair, and although I pick up some confusion about why I only use it sometimes, this is not universal. So maybe I'll get over these feelings in time.

In spite of my problems with the social model of disability, it has made a great difference to me. When I first became really ill with ME, I had many problems. I viewed them as the inevitable consequence of the illness, and as the illness went on and on, I felt more and more hopeless. The social model of disability taught me that things which seem tragic and inevitable are not necessarily so. I began to think more clearly about my problems and about what could be changed. It wasn't easy: I often had to settle for an inadequate substitute for something I had lost. But gradually, I have been able to remove some of my problems, and that gives me the hope that I need to survive.

Notes
1. ME Association Newsletter, Winter 1989, p. 36.
2. For fuller discussion of the social model see *Disabling Barriers – Enabling Environments*, ed. John Swain et al, (Resources List Part Four C); and 'Including All of Our Lives: Renewing the Social Model of Disability' by Liz Crow in *Encounters With Strangers*, ed. Jenny Morris (Resources List Part Four C).
3. For example in the introduction to *Encounters With Strangers*, and the article by Liz Crow mentioned in 2. above. *Lives Worth Living*, ed. Veronica Marris, covers the experiences of women with illnesses (Resources List Part Four C).
4. 'Disability, Impairment or Something In Between?' by Sally French in *Disabling Barriers – Enabling Environments*, op. cit.

The Paralympics

Kate Cook

Watching the paralympics on television filled me with such conflicting emotions. I cried with pride for the achievements of those athletes, but then I expect I'm not alone in that.

I watched and swung, like a pendulum. One moment thinking, 'well, I don't have a disability, not like these people. I can . . . and that's where I'd get stuck. Because I can, some days, do most things – that aren't too heavy, or don't involve too many stairs, or too far to walk.

But then, when the illness catches up with me again (which is always when I've got to thinking that maybe this time I'm nearly better), then, I can't. I can't go out, I can't think clearly enough to drive and I don't want to get up out of bed. I can't communicate; I'm in a bubble, where I know I ought to feel, but can't quite work out what.

Or then, I may just feel, have feelings for no good reason, cry and cry and cry, for nothing.

Talking this over with a friend who also has ME it became clear that it would be very hard to think of a paralympic sport for people with ME. Perhaps, we decided, it could be the Getting Out of Bed medal.

And it would be quite random who won, because it would just depend, on whatever it is that makes the difference (answers on a postcard please . . .).

But, whoever it was that won, the rest of us would be very pleased for them, because we would know how amazing that is, how wonderful those days are. Those days, when you can.

Beyond Convention

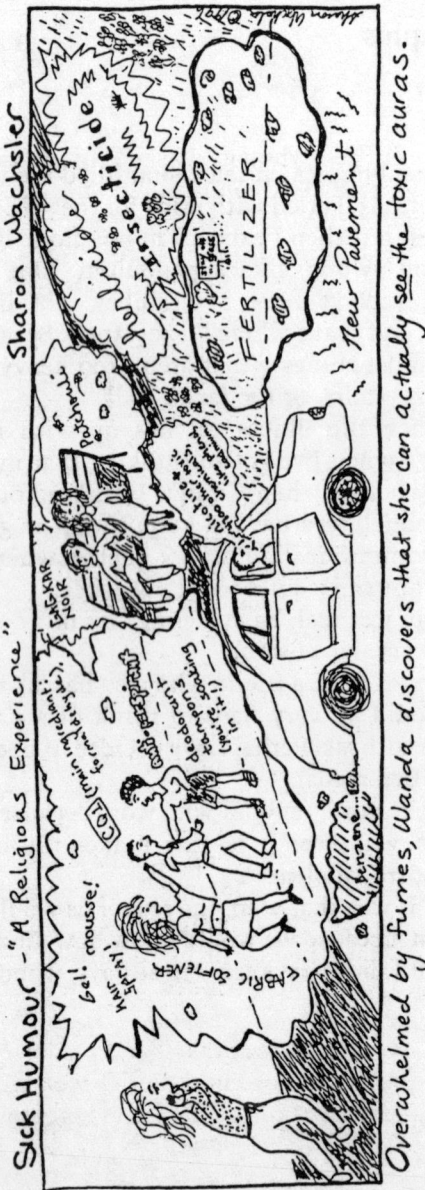

Introduction

Caeia March

In this final part of the anthology, I asked three practitioners who have been working with women who have ME, to write about the possibilities of healing from within their specialisms. Thus in this section it is the words of women working beyond conventional medicine that we read, rather than the voices of those who have ME.

This change of voice, a deliberate departure from the main theme of the anthology, has arisen in answer to the very many women with ME who, over the years, have mentioned that they are not confident to try this or that practice, because they don't really understand 'how it works'.

I chose to include the three that most often have been requested. I hope that the clarification may help some readers. I asked each practitioner to outline the theory behind her work, and to give us some direct examples of the way that her specialism might be applied to ME.

Herbal medicine and Chinese medicine have been with us for thousands of years. Homeopathy is younger, having been developed in the eighteenth century. These three healing practices are based on the assumption that the body has an innate ability to heal itself. When this ability is hidden, lost or damaged, its recovery can be enhanced once again. But there are no miracle cures, or quick fixes, and self-application is not advisable – including use of herbs, where long-term use should be monitored and dosage varies according to individual need. Further details of how to find a reliable and qualified practitioner may be found in the Resources List.

It can also be mentioned that any readers who are interested in other less well-known or newer remedies or treatments for ME will find interesting personal accounts and anecdotes in the journals of the ME Association and Action for ME. Remedies and fashions will come and go as we get to know ME and understand more about ourselves as women with ME.

I chose not to include any of the current fashions in healing in this section. As Shelley points out elsewhere, some of them are little understood or ineptly applied and we are right to be wary. Not so with herbal medicine, homeopathy and Chinese medicine. How they work has long been understood; how the woman with ME can respond to them is a developing field of knowledge for practitioners at present. These articles are therefore a sharing of old wisdom applied with great care to a new context: the context of ME.

Homeopathy and ME

Fiona D'Alwis

Hompeopathy offers a safe and rational alternative to conventional medicines: it aims to encourage and enhance our ability to heal ourselves, is suitable for both recent and long-standing conditions, and its effects are gentle and deep-acting. The approach is holistic: homeopaths take into account a person's mental, emotional and physical state, as well as the symptoms of the complaint, to select the remedy that will best stimulate their self-healing ability. Illness is not seen as just the sum total of recognised uniform symptoms; labelling a condition in this limited way means the individual's responses are lost, and their needs go unrecognised.

The main principle of homeopathy, and the one from which its name is derived, is the 'law of similars'. Symptoms produced during an illness are the individual's response to the state of disease. The symptoms result from the self-healing ability (conventionally described as the immune system) striving to restore balance, to bring about a return to health. For example, one reason for the rise in body temperature as a result of microbial infection is because this speeds up the metabolism, thereby increasing the activity of the white blood cells which destroy the microbes. In a fever case, therefore, a homeopath would prescribe a remedy that in a healthy person would produce a fever, thus assisting the body's self-healing process.

Jane's experience illustrates some aspects of homeopathic treatment.

Jane's Story, Part One

Jane is in her early twenties. Her first appointment is in August 1996, three months after being diagnosed with ME, although she had been experiencing severe symptoms since the previous winter. She had left college, found a job and bought a house in a short space of time. The work was 'hard going' with a 'vile' atmosphere in the office and her skills and abilities went unrecognised. Despite these stresses she continued at work because of financial commitments.

The long workdays, up to 70 hours weekly during the Christmas rush, took their toll, and she finally had to take sick leave after struggling with a constant cold and fainting several times. She tried to return after a month's rest but her symptoms soon worsened. Various medicines were prescribed including Prozac, vitamin supplements and analgesics, with limited relief.

One marked physical symptom is the recent pain in her legs that feels 'like acid rather than blood in my veins'. She cannot walk any distance and often uses a walking stick. She has had various sinus and allergy problems which have led to respiratory difficulties. She feels extremely tired and weak and has insomnia. She has also been much more emotional.

Mental work has never been a problem for her, but now her memory is poor, and at times she is unable to get her words out, they 'jumble into a mess, it's very frustrating'.

After college Jane returned to live in the same town as her parents and, although an only child, she has a very close extended family. She would prefer to be more independent.

In the last two years she has lost three close relatives and feels 'scared of losing anyone else'.

A Homeopathic Perspective

As a homeopath I try to have no assumptions about the illness or the person. What I am interested in is the individual's distinguishing symptoms or responses, and these are what I use to choose their most similar remedy. The common symptoms of ME which Jane suffers, such as extreme tiredness, are not as significant in this respect as the pain in her legs and the fainting episodes. As Jane had respiratory problems before ME they will take longer to clear than more recent symptoms. Her mental and emotional responses, especially to current stresses, are also considered in selecting a remedy; I particularly take into account her recent grief. (Stress refers to any external factor, such as exposure to viral or bacterial infection, chemicals and medicines including vaccinations, as well as physical and emotional trauma, which has an effect on well-being.)

When a person becomes ill, becomes out of balance, a healthy response is one that rapidly restores the balance. This response produces the symptoms which the patient feels and the homeopath can observe. These symptoms are not the illness, but rather the individual's response to the original state of imbalance. They are an indication of how deeply the person has been affected, or how far out of balance they are.

People vary and their responses to the same stress will also vary, which means that treatment has to be prescribed specifically for that person. Take, for example, exposure to a flu virus. One person may be unaffected because they are not susceptible. Another develops a high fever, and perhaps other symptoms, which last 24 hours as the body fights off the infection; after a day of rest they are well again. Someone else may develop a fever, but instead of feeling better after a few days they continue to suffer with lesser symptoms such as a cough, runny nose, sinusitis, headaches or tiredness which last several weeks. For yet another person this feeling of weakness after the flu may develop into more serious symptoms, such as recurring bronchitis or exhaustion, perhaps leading to feelings of inadequacy and depression as a result.

Acute and Chronic Diseases

Whether in acute (short) illness or chronic (long-standing) disease it is important to remember that the symptoms produced are the individual's best attempt at self-healing. If a person recovers with minimal disturbance there is obviously no need for treatment. However, when the physical symptoms persist, or even move on to an emotional or mental level, then homeopathic treatment can help.

In an acute illness there is often a clear causation. A healthy person will experience marked changes from normal, the differences called symptoms. Acute illnesses are often self-limiting and, with rest and good nutrition, the individual will usually recover. A homeopathic remedy can help to speed up the process.

In a chronic condition this attempt at self-healing has been unsuccessful. The person has been in a state of dis-ease for a while, and has become somewhat adapted to this decreased level of health. The initial cause may be less clear, and various triggers can easily exacerbate their condition. A thorough case history will reveal points where an inadequate response to a stress resulted in further depletion.

ME is an example of a chronic disease. There may be a clear trigger of an acute illness, but the individual may also describe having pushed themselves quite hard and struggled with, or perhaps even enjoyed, more than their share of challenging situations before their illness. Once the disease develops they are dramatically weakened. However, this lack of energy and strength is not easily measurable. The many combinations of symptoms, often seeming to encompass several different illnesses, makes ME confusing for those who need to name a disease before they can treat it. Orthodox medicine for a long time did not accept ME, often labelling such a variety of conditions as psychosomatic. Even today there are doctors and specialists who are unable to diagnose ME because there are no laboratory tests to 'prove' its existence.

All this has a bearing on the ME patient. If she has suffered with the condition for many years she may have had to put up with a lack of support from her doctor, and sometimes even disbelief from friends and family. This can further accentuate the isolation and loneliness that illness can provoke. A newly diagnosed patient may benefit from some legitimacy now that their symptoms have a name. However, along with the label come various preconceptions, including attitudes towards recovery times and treatment strategies, that can lead to feelings of impatience or despair.

The orthodox approach, with its many specialisations, can result in knowing more and more about less and less. It treats conditions with a standardised range of medicines: analgesics for joint pains, sedatives for insomnia, anti-depressants for depression, the list goes on. As a consequence of this approach someone who happens to have debilitating aches and pains and sleeplessness resulting in depression may end up taking several different medicines. This can mask the symptoms that are signalling the actual state of dis-ease; the person may think they are cured while the underlying problem remains. Homeopathy attends to the whole person, recognising their symptoms as an expression of their whole being, and seeks to go to the root of the patient's condition.

Jane's Story, Part Two

I see Jane again four weeks later. The pains in her legs have completely gone, but her sinus problems have worsened. Several new stresses have arisen to do with finances and relationships, more than one would ordinarily have to cope with. There is also a family holiday planned for the following month and, while having decided to use a wheelchair when necessary, Jane is still concerned not to spoil it for the others.

For some people an aggravation of some symptoms is not unusual in homeopathic treatment. Long-standing conditions can worsen as the vitality is increased, especially if symptoms have been controlled using conventional medication. It is a curative response, although most people regard it as a mixed blessing. Over time these older symptoms will also improve.

The Principles of Homeopathy

In homeopathy a remedy is given that produces symptoms in a healthy person similar to those expressed by the sick individual needing that particular remedy. For example, peeling an onion at first makes your nose tingle and your eyes water profusely. If you observe closely you notice that the discharge from the nose makes the skin sore while that from the eyes is bland. There is also a lot of sneezing. These are quite common symptoms at the beginning of a cold or hay fever for some people. Both of these conditions may be cured by the remedy Allium cepa (the onion), providing it is the most similar match with the person's other characteristic symptoms.

The founder of modern homeopathy was Samuel Hahnemann, although the idea of treating 'like with like' is ancient. Hahnemann (1755–1843) qualified as a doctor, but then gave up medicine because he felt that the treatments of the time were cruel. Rather than assisting the healing process these treatments weakened the already exhausted patients, resulting in further suffering, often compounded by drug-induced conditions. Instead Hahnemann became a translator and, in the course of this work, came across a piece by Dr William Cullen about the use of cinchona bark in the treatment of malaria. Cullen suggested that this substance worked because of its bitter and astringent taste. Hahnemann was also studying botany and chemistry and knew of other substances that had similar properties – and yet which had no effect on malarial fever. He decided to experiment on himself and took some cinchona, thereby bringing on symptoms similar to those of malaria; these symptoms continued for as long as he took the substance. This was his first proof of the law of similars.

Hahnemann spent several years testing other vegetable, mineral and animal substances on himself and colleagues. The testing of a substance is always carried out on human volunteers and is called a proving. Each substance produces a unique set of symptoms. Hahnemann also researched the medical records for the symptoms of accidental poisonings. All these sets of symptoms became the first *Materia Medica*, the homeopathic encyclopedia of remedies. Since then over two thousand other substances have been added to our books, and many have been retested to confirm the original findings.

A homeopathic prescription will consist of a single remedy, most closely matched to the person's condition. As the individual's symptoms change different remedies may be prescribed, but always singly. If remedies are combined their effects become unknowable and this can confuse the case.

Another important principle is that of the minimum dose. Homeopathic remedies contain the tiniest amount of the material substance. They are therefore unbelievably dilute, but at the same time their strength or potency is maintained. This is because homeopathic remedies seek to stimulate the person's self-healing capacity dynamically. The effects of the correctly chosen remedy can be profound and very long lasting; it may be months before another remedy is needed. As well as experiencing an amelioration of their original symptoms a person will often say that after taking the remedy they experienced a general increase in that immeasurable quality, 'well-being'.

Jane's Story, Continued

Because of the holiday I do not see Jane again for seven weeks. She describes the break as 'brilliant' and, although she has spent much time in the wheelchair, she is walking further than previously, and managed the last holiday dance with her mother. Standing for any length of time is still tiring, and she feels that because the past week has been particularly busy she has become too exhausted and 'shaky' at times. Other signs that she may have overdone things include dizziness, sensitivity to noise and increased perspiration, all useful indicators to take things easier for a while. She realises she will have to listen to her body and stop when these symptoms appear, acknowledging her needs and frustrations when this happens, which is no mean task. The sinus symptoms improved after the remedy but are gradually worsening again.

Our fourth appointment is another seven weeks later. Jane has recently been experiencing strange temperature fluctuations, one moment very cold and needing to be wrapped up, at other times surprisingly warm. Of greater concern are her financial problems. She values her independence highly, although living alone has been a bit of a strain. She tries to put a brave face on things but the effort is telling. She has been busy making Christmas presents and cards. In addition she has been doing word-processing and typing at college, with examinations coming up in the new year. Work prospects in the area are limited and these added skills will widen her options; she is also prepared to consider moving away if necessary. What she is clear about is that she doesn't want anything 'too high-pressured'.

I am concerned about Jane's emotional and mental stance: being one of life's copers she is used to making light of her discomfort, but is now 'running out of jokes'. While it isn't helpful to dwell on one's condition, reflection can lead to realisation of what is really causing the distress and this acknowledgement creates the confidence to adapt and change. Jane's view that 'the perseverance factor is strong in women' may make it difficult for her to spend time valuing and looking after herself. This is true for many of us. Of course practical necessities also push us to override these instinctive responses, and personality and upbringing have a part to play as well.

Over the winter Jane's progress is set back when she develops new symptoms, as a result of a flu epidemic in the area. She moves into her parents' home for the duration (three weeks), but feels disappointed with herself. My experience of this particular epidemic is that many people who consider themselves healthy have taken time to get over it, and three weeks is not unreasonable for her. The symptoms she experienced were strong, unlike anything she has experienced in years. This usually indicates a dynamic self-healing capacity in an acute illness. I interpret Jane's symptoms to be the result of her strengthened immune system successfully responding to an infection, rather than a relapse of her ME. This is borne out by her continued improvement in February and March.

On another positive note, she sat one of her exams before

succumbing to the illness, and has been helping her mother out with some household chores, which has enabled her to feel better about herself. However, she expresses a despondency, lack of assertiveness and feelings of being overwhelmed, which call for another remedy. In her own words, 'I need a goal, and I don't have one.'

An individual operates as a whole or integrated totality which is greater than the sum of the parts. Homeopathy maintains that there is a governing dynamic force that enables a person to operate in this way. It is expressed in various philosophies as the spirit, vital force, chi, prana or energy. In illness it is this energy that prompts the expression of symptoms. In health it is this same energy that seeks to free us from the limits of our (perceived) inadequacies.

From Great Abyss to Gate of Hope:
An Exploration of the Treatment of ME by Traditional Chinese Medicine

Kate Wilson

Linda teaches in an infant school. She came for acupuncture because for six months her energy had been very low. She complained of heavy aching legs, of feeling cold and of being unable to think clearly. After eating she could barely stay awake and it was becoming hard to do her job well. She had been off work several times in the last year with a sore throat and swollen glands which she was never able to completely shake off.

June had been ill for five years. Her main symptoms were complete exhaustion, constipation, backache, frequent urination at night and a tendency to catch colds. Her sleep patterns were completely disrupted and although she was very tired she often felt agitated and restless. She had no recollection of an infection prior to the onset of ME but had taken many courses of antibiotics for chest infections in her early twenties.

Both these women are fictitious, though their case histories are based on my experiences of treating women with ME.

Traditional Chinese Medicine has been practised for over 2,000 years. It is based on a philosophy of life which views the universe as a living dynamic organism. The energy which flows through the cosmos is called Qi (pronounced chee). The concept of Qi is central to Chinese Medicine and it is important to explain it before going on to describe diagnosis and treatment. Qi may be defined as 'life force', and wherever there is life there is Qi. It is the basic stuff of life – present within us and in the whole world around us including the mountains and the oceans. The movement and flow of Qi creates the seasons, the weather, the thoughts in our minds and the feelings in our hearts. Chinese Medicine aims to work with the flow of Qi. Perhaps without knowing it we may recognise within ourselves the flow of Qi energy: some days we feel heavy and depressed – the Qi is stagnant. Then something mysteriously lifts and our mood changes – Qi is moving smoothly again.

Seasonal changes reflect the movement of Qi and each season is linked with particular organs. In spring Qi is rising like the sap in the trees. This time is associated with the Liver and if the liver energy is unwell then the spring may be a difficult time. In summer the Qi is expansive and abundant. The trees are in full leaf and people seem more warm, relaxed and friendly. This is the time associated with the Heart. In late summer there is the harvest, a time of collecting and gathering which is linked to the energies of the Stomach and Spleen. In autumn the Qi begins to withdraw and return to the earth for the winter rest. This can be a time of grief, the emotion associated with the Lungs and Intestines. People who are not in tune with this season may find it hard to slow down and may exhaust themselves if they are unable to find a way to relax. In winter the Qi resides deep in the earth, lying dormant in the roots of the trees. It is a natural time for rest and reflection. The complexities and stresses of our world can make it difficult to connect with these natural cycles but perhaps this is one of the great challenges of our time. According to the principles of Chinese Medicine we must follow the guidelines provided by the seasons if we are to maintain health. As women we are also attuned to lunar cycles of Qi which affect our fertility, creativity and emotions. There is also a daily pattern of Qi ebbing and flowing which is mirrored in our need for periods of activity and rest. In ME these natural rhythms are often disrupted giving symptoms such as sleep disturbance, breathing difficulty, inability to recover after exertion and a deep feeling of being 'at odds' within the self.

In western medicine ME has been controversial in terms of

its cause, its diagnosis and its treatment. The naming of the disease has reflected some of these problems, ranging from the highly medical Myalgic Encephalomyelitis to the simply derogatory 'yuppie flu'. Chinese Medicine has not been faced with these problems. The signs and symptoms of ME, however varied and wide ranging, can be approached in the usual way – interpreted, diagnosed and treated according to ancient principles. These principles are based on a wealth of knowledge that has been well documented, researched and practised for hundreds of years. Chinese Medicine includes the therapies of acupuncture, moxibustion (warming the energy by burning a dried herb above or on the skin), Chinese herbalism and advice on diet and lifestyle. It would be better named Oriental Medicine as it is a system of medicine practised in many countries including China, Japan, Vietnam and Korea. In the West we draw from all these different sources, thus enriching our practice, but this also means that the treatment received may differ from one practitioner to the next. There is no one approach to the treatment of ME by a practitioner of Chinese Medicine although certain basic principles will be shared by all. If seeking treatment I would advise you to:

  i) Check that the practitioner is registered with the British Acupuncture Council;
 ii) Find someone you feel comfortable with;
iii) Ask them about their approach and how they will work with you.

A question that is commonly asked is 'Can acupuncture help ME?' The simple answer is 'yes', and evidence from research backs this up. However, the question comes from a western perspective. Acupuncture is a person-centred treatment rather than a disease-centred one. There may be some similarities in the treatment of different people with ME, but there is always an individual treatment plan based on the diagnosis of the whole person – body, mind, emotions and spirit. The diagnosis is made by looking at the person, listening to their story and asking questions about personal and medical history. In addition the pulse is taken on the wrists, the tongue is examined closely for its shape, markings and coating, and some practitioners also feel the abdomen, looking for areas of discomfort, strength and weakness. The practitioner will be seeking answers to the following questions: What is the state of this person's Qi? What has happened to disrupt the flow? What are the strengths within her that can be used to promote self-healing?

Gradually a picture forms of the disharmony which is leading to illness or dis-ease. This picture will be the starting point for a journey of discovery for both client and practitioner. The discussions that are sparked off by the Chinese diagnosis often play a major part in the healing process.

Qi is further described as relating specifically to different organs, but the word organ means much more than in western medicine. In Chinese Medicine the terms Liver, Spleen, Heart, etc. refer to a whole system of energy as well as the actual organ. An imbalance in the Liver Qi will at first only affect the energy flow. This subtle imbalance can be detected early on from symptoms such as headaches, painful breasts or blurred vision and it will also show up in the pulse and on the tongue. Deterioration of the actual organ is the result of prolonged and severe imbalance and may never occur. To describe this further I will take the example of the Spleen because there is often a problem with the Qi of the Spleen when someone has ME.

As I mentioned earlier, the Spleen and its related organ the Stomach are closely connected with the season of late summer – a time of harvest and celebration. Other associations with Spleen/Stomach energy are the colour yellow, the emotion of sympathy, the sound of singing and the element Earth. The Spleen's main functions in Chinese Medicine are to transform food and drink into pure Qi and then to transport this vital energy to all parts of the body. Common problems arising from dysfunction of this system are tiredness (insufficient Qi is being taken to the body especially the arms and legs), digestive problems (the transformation process has broken down) and accumulation of fluids leading to swelling, heavy sluggish feelings, a muggy head and lack of ability to think clearly. As you may remember, many of these problems had arisen for Linda.

An important principle in Chinese Medicine is that a small part can reflect the state of the whole. The pulse and the tongue diagnosis can give as much information as several hours of talking. The pulse is felt on the radial artery of each wrist and gives detailed information about the state of the Qi and of the internal organs. For example, the pulse of the Liver is found on the left wrist. The practitioner notes the speed but is equally interested in the quality of the pulse. Is it weak and faltering, taut like a guitar string or steady and calm? June's Kidney pulse was very weak but this did not mean there was a serious problem with her actual Kidney organs.

The condition of the tongue is also an indicator of the health of the whole person. Linda had a pale tongue showing a deficiency in her vital energy. It was also wet with a white coat, showing the accumulation of fluids in her body.

The treatment follows on from the diagnosis. Chinese herbs are commonly used in conjunction with acupuncture, and this combination has proved most effective in the treatment of ME. However, for the purposes of this article I intend to focus on acupuncture – the use of needles.

Acupuncture points are found on the surface of the body on pathways of energy which have been documented for thousands of years. No one knows how or when they were originally discovered, but with centuries of use detailed knowledge has accumulated about the healing potential of each point. Most people want to know, 'Will it hurt when the needles are put in?' It is helpful to imagine the points as openings to the deeper energy. When the practitioner is skilful and the client is relaxed the needle should go in quite painlessly. Needles are then manipulated slightly to make contact with the Qi: this can and should produce a sensation such as an ache or a tingle. In a single treatment 4 to 12 needles may be used. They may be taken out immediately or left in for 15–20 minutes, and during this time many people take the opportunity to relax and focus on themselves. Commonly, people fall asleep or go into a deep meditative rest.

It is not possible to say how many treatments will be needed. Even when many of the symptoms have cleared, the underlying energy is usually still weak and to avoid a relapse the treatments must continue in order to nourish the Qi. Initially sessions are weekly, becoming less frequent as the Qi strengthens. ME is typically a 'two steps forward and one step back' illness and although benefits are experienced from the start, the long-term recovery is not fast and patience is needed. Acupuncture works on emotional and spiritual levels as well as the physical and can be a great support in times of distress. There is a point on the Liver pathway called *Gate of Hope* which reminds us that hope is always there but sometimes we forget to open the gate.

With the additional insights Chinese Medicine can offer it should be possible to closely monitor the state of your own Qi. If an acute illness threatens then immediate treatment can keep it at bay. There is an ancient Chinese text devoted to the study of the different stages of acute diseases which has proved very useful in the diagnosis and treatment of ME. It is important to know when to clear an infection and when to strengthen the Qi. The practitioner must be attuned to the progression of the illness and give appropriate treatment. Herbs specifically to deal with colds and flu can be kept at home for use when needed. The Qi is nourished by regular acupuncture treatment and by paying serious attention to maintaining life-enhancing rhythms. Chinese Medicine stresses the importance of developing routines in everyday life and this particularly applies to people with ME. This means listening to your rhythms and knowing what pattern will suit you best. It is important to establish a regular bedtime and if possible have a rest in the afternoon. Regular meals eaten in a relaxed and unhurried manner allow the stomach time to digest and nourish the Spleen Qi. A simple meditation technique such as focusing on the breath can also help to draw attention to an inner rhythm that is always present.

I shall now discuss in more depth the diagnosis and treatment of Linda and June.

Linda's symptoms show a weakness in the Spleen energy. The Qi is cold and weak, allowing a build-up of dampness in her system. Damp is heavy and tends to settle in the lower half of the body leading to symptoms such as aching legs. Because the Spleen takes energy all over the body her head also feels foggy and unclear. For Linda life felt like a permanent wet dreary afternoon. She was lethargic, depressed and found it difficult to motivate herself. Weak Spleen energy gives rise to digestive problems and Linda's food sat in a heavy lump in her stomach making her feel tired and sleepy. Linda reported that she had been ill for six months. Prior to this she had an immunisation which in Chinese Medicine is comparable to an infection and she never quite recovered from it. Her energy was already depleted from long working hours and many years of poor diet. She had no regular routines in her life and was never able to catch up on the rest she needed.

There was another factor in Linda's history which may have weakened the Spleen energy. Linda's mother died when she was very young and she grew up in a children's home. In Chinese Medicine the Spleen is associated with the mother principle and the ability to nourish the self. Early difficulties in life make an impression on our patterns of energy. Acupuncture is able to work deeply on emotional and spiritual levels, and specific points on the Stomach and Spleen pathways were used to help Linda heal past hurts. These points have names which give us clues to their healing potential. *Heavenly Pivot* helped Linda find her own spiritual centre. *Abdomen Sorrow* encouraged the release of tears. *Great Welcome* helped her feel entitled to be here.

Chinese Medicine does not separate the physical from the emotional and spiritual as we are accustomed to in the West, and all aspects of the person's life are considered equally important. This is a major difference between the western and the oriental approaches as our society exaggerates the importance of physical symptoms which can be measured scientifically and tends to dismiss the emotional and spiritual ones. Most people with ME have been told at some time that their symptoms are not 'real' and that it is 'all in the mind'. Chinese Medicine views ME as a disharmony of the Qi energy which has arisen from the weaving together of many different factors, physical, emotional and spiritual, and symptoms would be expected to manifest on all these levels.

Linda's early experience made it hard for her to ask for help and it was an important step to come for acupuncture. Gradually her body gained strength and she experienced a growing sense of well-being which helped her through the inevitable ups and downs of recovery. She developed routines of self-care and created a rhythm in her daily life which allowed her to follow her energy fluctuations rather than fight against them.

Many of June's symptoms were similar to Linda's but there was a different pattern of disharmony underlying her illness. Weak Kidney Qi was indicated by urinary problems, back pain and a deep exhaustion. The Kidneys are easily weakened by overwork and especially by too much standing. As a young teenager June helped on a market stall, standing for long hours often in bad weather. Long-term use of antibiotics had further weakened her immune system. In her thirties she worked for several years as a laboratory technician in a photographic studio and repeated exposure to toxic chemicals had worsened her condition. As well as acupuncture and herbs to build up the Kidney Qi she was advised to rest in the afternoon. There is a time of day associated with each organ, and for the Kidneys and Bladder this is the afternoon, when there is greater potential for healing. June also began to take more care of her lower back by keeping it warm, avoiding draughts and becoming aware of the need to relax when she was lifting or carrying heavy loads. She also took up meditation and found the breathing exercises helped her to slow down. June often breathed only using her upper chest and this was adding to her feelings of anxiety. The strengthening of her Kidney Qi helped bring the breath down deeper into her abdomen and gave her a new sense of being rooted and safe. Winter is the season associated with the Kidneys, and during those months June made a special effort to seek out quiet space for reflection and rest. Acupuncture points such as *Sea of Qi*, *Great Abyss* and *Greater Mountain Stream* helped to replenish her own inner reserves of energy.

Traditional Chinese Medicine is an ideal form of treatment for diseases of the immune system such as ME because it has the capacity not only to clear infections but also to strengthen the underlying energy. Treatments are based on a thorough understanding of the whole person, taking into account their strengths and weaknesses. However, it is what happens in the rest of our lives that holds the key to recovery. Even with no acupuncture at hand we may all benefit from paying attention to the seasons, listening to the rhythm of the Qi within us and living in harmony with natural cycles of rest and activity.

Bibliography
Hill, Sandra, 'A Discussion of two cases of ME', *European Journal of Oriental Medicine* Vol. 1, No. 3, Spring 1994.
De Soriano, Gretchen, 'ME – A Japanese Perspective', *European Journal of Oriental Medicine* Vol. 1, No. 4, Autumn 1994.
Maciocia, Giovanni, 'Myalgic Encephalomyelitis', *The Journal of Chinese Medicine*, No. 35, Jan. 1991.

Herbs and ME

Niki Green

Herbs have much to offer in aiding recovery from ME. Increasingly the work of the modern herbalist is with chronic diseases like ME where a broad restorative approach is required. Most importantly herbal treatment for ME aims to encourage the body's self-healing abilities – what used to be called the vital force. So the medicinal plants used are gentle, non-toxic and safe for use over a number of months. We know now that there is no one cause and no one magic solution to ME, so a holistic approach emphasises that herbs should be taken in conjunction with plenty of rest, a good wholesome (preferably additive-free) diet and a positive mental outlook.

The range of plant medicines available is enormous and using them most effectively requires experience and expertise. Self-healing is certainly possible with herbs, using only very safe and gentle medicines, some of which I describe in this article, but there is a strong case for consulting a properly trained and qualified herbal practitioner. A professional medical herbalist will take a detailed case history concerning the individual's medical history, current health problems, diet, lifestyle and constitution before making a prescription which may include quite a number of different herbs and is specifically tailored to the needs of the individual. Members of the National Institute of Medical Herbalists have undergone a thorough four-year theoretical and practical training before joining the Institute and starting a practice.

The herbal approach begins with the central feature of the illness – extreme fatigue. This fatigue is a clear indication that the body's vital reserves are severely depleted. It seems probable that whatever the specific trigger of the illness –

whether environmental pollutants or one of the many different viruses which have been implicated – many sufferers were already stressed to a point where they were unable to deal with the challenge to their immune systems. It is interesting to note in this context that in the well-known outbreak of the disease in 1955 at the Royal Free Hospital in London, those who succumbed were overwhelmingly the staff, busy people with stressful jobs who, unlike the patients, were unable to rest and recuperate. In the same way, mothers of young children are known to be a high risk category because not only are they exposed to many of the enteroviruses known to act as triggers for the illness, but they are less able than most people to rest and recover properly from a viral infection. Unfortunately once someone has contracted ME they often have disturbed sleep patterns and wake still tired even after long periods of sleep, so a first aim of treatment is to improve this situation. There are many herbal relaxants and nervous system restoratives which can be employed for this purpose. The first principle of prescribing (even more importantly in self-prescribing by an untrained person) is to use the gentlest of remedies first and allow them enough time, possibly several weeks, to become effective. Chamomile (*Matricaria recutita*) and lemon balm (*Melissa officinalis*) are both good examples of gentle, safe relaxants which are also useful for calming an upset digestion. Either of these may be drunk as a tea (one teaspoon of dried herb per cup) and should be drunk during the day as well as before bedtime. Lime or linden flowers (*Tilia europea*) are slightly stronger but still perfectly safe for everyday use and very appropriate where there is a lot of nervous irritability accompanying sleep disturbance.

Valerian (*Valeriana officinalis*) is an effective tranquillising plant remedy but is best used as part of a balanced prescription from a professional herbalist. Warm baths before bedtime are relaxing in themselves but the effect can be heightened with the use of a few drops of essential oil. It has been shown that essential oils inhaled in steam – as in a bath – are absorbed directly into the limbic system of the brain which plays an important part in balancing our emotions. I would particularly recommend good quality lavender oil for its relaxing and soothing qualities. In addition to calming herbal baths and bedtime drinks it is important to learn how to relax properly in a situation where sound sleep is so vital to recovery, so I would suggest trying out one or two of the many relaxation tapes commercially available. There are different styles to suit different personality types so it should be possible to find one that suits with a little perseverance. Another possibility is to consult a hypnotherapist who can teach relaxation by auto-suggestion or make a tape tailored to the individual.

Sufferers from Chronic Fatigue Syndrome often describe the emotional instability which accompanies it – expressed as dramatic mood swings, acute sensitivity, anxiety and depression. It is probably impossible to differentiate between the factors that cause this – how much the nervous debility is part of the illness and how much is consequent upon the effects the illness is having on the person's life – but there are various herbal remedies which can help. The calming herbs discussed already clearly have a part to play, but there are two others that I would recommend as nervine restoratives. The first is oatstraw (*Avena sativa*) which may be obtained in the form of a tincture. Little in the way of research appears to have been done on the action of this plant, but herbalists regard it as a specific restorative for nervous exhaustion and debility and essential to a programme of convalescence from any serious or chronic illness. Both anxiety and depression may be helped by this remedy. The seed may be used in the same way, taken in the form of oatmeal. Organic oatmeal porridge (made in the normal way) eaten every morning will stabilise blood sugar levels and is one of the most simple and useful self-help measures for nervous exhaustion. The second herb I find invaluable in treatment is St John's wort (*Hypericum perforatum*), which may be also obtained in tincture form. This is useful for any condition involving nervous tension and seems to help both anxiety and mild depression. Like

Avena, it is a relaxant and also acts to reduce pain; those suffering from the illness often find that muscle and joint pains respond favourably to this herb. Another herb traditionally used to lift the spirits (probably best used in the form of essential oil) is rosemary. This, used like lavender oil in the bath, is often surprisingly effective in improving 'low' moods, relieving headaches and achieving mental alertness for a time. Rosemary oil may also be used on its own or as an ingredient in a rubbing oil for external use in painful areas. It helps to relieve muscle and nerve pain and stimulate circulation. The oil should always be diluted at least 1:10 in a base vegetable oil (e.g. almond, olive or sunflower) before use on the skin.

Turning to the treatment of more deep-seated aspects of the illness, there are a few herbs I have found to be particularly useful. Firstly, echinacea (*Echinacea angustifolium* and *purpureum*). This is a North American plant in the same family as rudbeckia – often grown as an ornamental in gardens. It was traditionally used by the native population for a wide range of infections and has a modern reputation for being useful in immunological disturbance and hypersensitivity reactions like allergies. There is evidence that it can be of use in viral as well as bacterial infections. With ME sufferers it may be that echinacea assists the body to finally resolve the viral infection which is so often the initial trigger for the illness and mediates inappropriate immune responses.

Secondly, research into ME has demonstrated disturbances in hypothalamic control which in turn affects the adrenal glands. Liquorice (*Glycyrrhiza glabra*) is one of the most widely used plant remedies in the world, and a lot of research has been undertaken to investigate its properties. It is used in many conditions but particularly those involving exaggerated inflammatory responses. ME sufferers have been shown to have lowered levels of cortisol, an anti-inflammatory steroidal hormone, which may contribute to an exaggeration of allergic responses and to the reactivation of dormant viruses. The glycosides in liquorice resemble the natural steroids present in the body and can be used to support the adrenals when under stress. It is often used as a classic 'tonic' herb, meaning it results in a general improvement in the capacity to handle all manner of stresses and return the body to balance. This broad restorative action makes it very suitable for aiding recovery from long-standing chronic illnesses where exhaustion and debility are prominent features. Liquorice is however a powerful remedy, despite its familiarity as a confection, and is best used with the supervision of a trained practitioner.

A particular problem for women with ME is that already existing problems relating to the menstrual cycle may worsen, or this may become a problem area, with the onset of the illness. The same disturbance of the hypothalamic pituitary functions which leads to adrenal imbalance also affects the ovaries and thus the hormones involved in the menstrual cycle. This is a complex area, again probably best treated by the professional herbalist, but hormonal balancing remedies such as helonias root (*Chamaelirium luteum*) and agnus castus (*Vitex agnus castus*) may be appropriate. Self-help is also possible with the use of dandelion (*Taraxacum*) root and/or leaf. This very safe remedy may be taken as a decoction (roots and barks are often taken in this way, involving the boiling of the herb in water for a few minutes) or a tea (in the case of the leaf) and has bitter and diuretic properties. Bitters stimulate liver function and thus assist the regulation of the levels of circulating hormones in the blood – breaking down and eliminating those that are excess to requirements. The diuretic action of the herb is useful for those who experience water retention – a common problem for women with ME. Another very safe bitter tonic herb which may be taken as a tea is English pot marigold or *Calendula*. This is also anti-fungal in its action and therefore of benefit to women with vaginal thrush or excessive candida albicans in the bowel. While the link between candida and ME is still disputed, the overgrowth of this yeast is certainly more common in anyone who has suffered from a chronic illness and is severely debilitated.

Finally it is worth considering taking a supplement of evening primrose oil combined with Vitamin E, which increases its effectiveness. This is generally a very safe supplement although it is not suitable for anyone with epilepsy. It is now well known for the relief of PMT symptoms, and clinical trials have also demonstrated that it can be as effective as orthodox anti-inflammatory drugs in relieving joint pain in arthritic conditions. It contains large amounts of an essential fatty acid which plays a part in prostaglandin metabolism – a very complex chemical pathway which underlies appropriate immune response – especially in mediating inflammation. In a 1990 clinical trial (quoted in *Living with ME* by Dr Charles Shepherd), ME sufferers taking this supplement experienced significant improvement in a range of symptoms.

Hopefully these brief notes give an indication of the many medicinal plants which may be useful in this debilitating condition. Consulting a professional practitioner and/or the use of the gentlest remedies in a positive self-help programme can be a big step forward on the road to recovery.

Resources List

In different articles throughout the anthology contributors have mentioned books or groups or remedies. We have collected the information here and listed it to match the four sections of the anthology. (Unless otherwise mentioned the phone numbers are for voice telephones.)

Part One: Diagnosis, Definitions and Decisions

ACTION FOR ME is a national membership organisation that offers help, information and other services to people with ME. Members receive three copies a year of the journal *Interaction*. Members also benefit from information and counselling helplines, postal libraries, welfare and legal advice services and a national network of local groups. For further information and details of membership please send a large s.a.e. to:
Action for ME, PO BOX 1302, Wells, Somerset BA5 2WE
tel: 01749 670799   fax: 01749 672561

ME ASSOCIATION
The ME Association exists to give support to all those affected by ME. The association is now a charitable trust and offers a wide range of services, including a quarterly membership magazine, *Perspectives*, informing and advising members.
Write to The ME Association, 4 Corringham Road, Stanford-le-Hope, Essex SS17 0AH
tel: 01375 642466   fax: 01375 360256

WESTCARE
Westcare is a registered charity set up in July 1989, which provides services for people with PVFS/ME/CFS. Its main clinic is in Bristol and provides consultations with professional

advisers/counsellors. Under the initiative of Westcare there has been published a Report of the National Task Force on CFS/PVFS/ME. This report costs £6.95 including p&p and has an invaluable overview of the history of ME; the definitions of the different terms and criteria for diagnosis; an appendix on diagnosis in children; an extensive reading list; and list of journal references. It is accessible in terms of plain English and extremely informative. Well worth the money.

Westcare is at 155 Whiteladies Road, Clifton, Bristol, BS8 2RF
tel: 0117 9239341   fax: 0117 9239347

NATIONAL ME SUPPORT CENTRE
This is a registered charity based within a National Health Service Trust. The centre offers medical and non-medical counselling for patients with a firm diagnosis of CFS/ME. It is linked to the medical and neurological clinics.

Address: Disablement Services Centre, Harold Wood Hospital, Romford, Essex RM3 9AR
tel: 01708 378050   fax: 01708 378032

Two general good background books, both written by GPs with first-hand information on ME, are recommended by several contributors.

Shepherd, Dr Charles, *Living with ME*, Cedar Books, 1992, ISBN 0 7493 1264 5.

MacIntyre, Dr Anne, *ME: How to live with it*, Thorsons, 1992, ISBN 0 7225 2642 5.

and for young people:

Moss, Jill I, *Somebody Help ME*, Sunbow Books, 1995, ISBN 0 9525 783 01.

New titles are being produced all the time as understanding of ME increases. Reviews can be found in the journals mentioned above.

Part Two: Family, Friends and Community

LOCAL ME GROUPS can be found from the ME Association and Action for ME. If you haven't got a group in your area and wish to start one, this can be done via the listings in the journals.

Contributors have sent in the following local information:

CALDER VALLEY DISABLED WOMEN'S NETWORK
The Calder Valley Disabled Women's Network exists for social contact, friendship, mutual support and information exchange. Any woman who considers herself as disabled or chronically sick for whatever reason is very welcome.
Contact June Eaton, Lower Crimsworth Cottage, Pecket Well, Hebden Bridge, West Yorks, HX7 8RB.
tel: 01422 844914. Phone calls after 4 pm please.

LEICESTER
Lesbian Gay and Bisexual Centre. It has a newsletter and several health projects.
15 Wellington Street, Leicester, LE1 6HH
tel: 0116 254 7412

MANCHESTER
The Pankhurst Centre is a women's centre with a newsletter.
60–62 Nelson Street, Manchester, M13
tel: 0161 273 5673
Eve's Back is Manchester women's quarterly networking magazine.
BOX 65, 1 Newton Street, Manchester, M1 1HW

NOTTINGHAM
The Women's Centre has many different groups and events.
30 Chaucer Street, Nottingham, NG1 5LP
tel: 0115 985 9862

NATIONAL CONTACTS AND GROUPS

ALTERNATIVES This is a mail order book service of second-hand books by and for women, with a good range of titles available on health and disability. New books can be ordered. Useful for women who are isolated for whatever

reason and cannot get to bookshops.
Send A5 s.a.e. for catalogue to:
49 Vyvyan Street, Cambourne, TR14 8AS
tel: 01209 716557

ASIAN WOMEN'S RESOURCE CENTRE
108 Craven Park, London, NW10
tel: 0181 961 5701/6549

AYME The Association of Youth with ME was founded in 1996
for young people with ME ages 5–25. There is a bi-monthly
magazine, plus a penpal service, phone contacts and postal
library.
PO BOX 605, Milton Keynes, MK6 3EX
tel: 01908 691635

BLACK WOMEN'S ACTION GROUP
76 Elsted Road, London, SE17
tel: 0171 708 1643

BLACK WOMEN'S MENTAL HEALTH PROJECT
12 Donovan Court, Exton Crescent, London, NW10
tel: 0181 961 6324

BOADICEA DISABLED WOMEN'S NEWSLETTER is published by the
Greater London Association of Disabled People, and is
available from GLAD, 336 Brixton Road, London, SW9 7AA
tel: 0171 346 5800   fax: 0171 346 5810
Boadicea is available in print, large print and on tape.

DISABILITY NOW This is a monthly magazine on rights,
information, debates and issues.
Published by SCOPE
12 Park Crescent, London, W1N 4EQ
tel: 0171 636 5020   fax: 0171 436 4582   minicom:
0171 436 9914

FROM THE FLAMES is a publication of radical feminism with
spirit, with current debates within women's politics
(including health), creativity, and spirituality. The magazine
takes an anti-racist and international approach. Write for

current publication schedules and more information to:
42 Mapperley Road, Nottingham, NG3 5AS

GEMMA is a national friendship and information network of lesbian and bisexual women, disabled and non-disabled, with a quarterly newsletter.
address: BM BOX 5700, London, WC1N 3XX

IRISH WOMEN'S CENTRE
59 Stoke Newington Church Street, London, N16
tel: 0171 249 7318

JEWISH ME GROUP This is part of the Action for ME organisation. Write for information and contact numbers to Action for ME.

KENRIC is a national social organisation for lesbians with a newsletter, contacts and social events. There are groups in most areas. Write for information with s.a.e. to:
BM Kenric, London, WC1N 3XX

LESBIAN ME NETWORK. This is a national network of support and friendship and will have a newsletter.
The contact number is Karon on 01933 383182

LESBIAN LINE LONDON operates from Monday to Friday 2–10 pm on 0171 251 6911. Although this is the London number you can ask for numbers for other areas from this number. An ansaphone will tell you if the times have had to be changed, and in case it's urgent, it gives the number of the Lesbian and Gay Switchboard.

MANGO SEASON is the magazine of the Caribbean Women Writers' Alliance and carries information on courses, events and groups. Available from the Caribbean Centre, Goldsmiths College, New Cross, London, SE14 6NW

PARENTABILITY
This is a national network of disabled people who are parents or hope to become parents. The network welcomes people with physical or sensory impairments, long-term illnesses and people with learning difficulties. Services are

also offered to professionals who work alongside disabled parents. Contact is via the National Childbirth Trust (NCT) office with 24-hour ansaphone. There is a network of local groups for advice on Pregnancy, Childbirth and Parenthood. It is run by volunteers working from home.
Write c/o NCT, Alexandra House, Oldham Terrace, Acton, London, W3 6NH
tel: 0181 992 2616

THE PINK PAPER This lesbian and gay newsletter has listings for all kinds of groups and carries classified ads for people wanting to start groups. It often has articles on health. People in isolated areas can have it posted.
Write to: 72 Holloway Road, London, N7 8NZ
tel: 0171 296 6000

SILVER MOON WOMEN'S BOOKSHOP
Mail order available and quarterly newsletter.
62–65 Charing Cross Road, London, WC1
tel: 0171 836 7906

TYMES (The Young ME Sufferer). This is an informative quarterly newsletter for young people with ME. It provides a phone and correspondence service for members and their carers/parents needing advice and support.
Write to: 9 Patching Hall Lane, Chelmsford, Essex, CM1 4DH
tel: 01245 263482

WOMEN MAKING A DIFFERENCE: A directory for Change. This new publication has been compiled by the erstwhile Everywoman group. It lists many kinds of women's organisations, centres, businesses, courses, groups and health projects. It is published by Feminist Publishing, ISBN 0952 9740 02

YOUNG PEOPLE – The ME Association is 'in the process of setting up committees to decide what kind of services the group wants to provide' (September 1997). Write for information to the ME Association.

Part Three: Healing Ourselves

These are the resources from Shelley's article:

• Jin Shin – Contact ASHM: ASSOCIATION OF SELF HELP MEDICINE on 01703 559008, or at 21 Harcourt Road, Bitterne Park, Southampton, SO18 1GQ.
• Sunrider herbs are available from ASHM, or ASHM can refer you direct to Sunrider.
• Nature's Own vitamin C – some health food shops stock this, or contact the manufacturer direct on 01684 310022.
• THE CINNAMON TRUST is a charity offering volunteers to care for your pet if you have to go into hospital. Tel: 01736 757900.
• BioCare, manufacturers of Mycopryl – contact them on 0121 433 3727, or write to them at Lakeside, 180 Lifford Lane, Kings Norton, Birmingham, B30 3NT. Try asking for a 10% discount; if not you could try ordering through Revital health shop, tel; 0181 459 3382 or freephone 0800 252875, at 35 High Road, Willesden, London, NW10 2TE.
• Linusit Gold cracked linseeds are available from most health food shops.
• NATIONAL FEDERATION OF SPIRITUAL HEALERS are on 01932 783164, or write to them at Old Manor Farm Studio, Church Street, Sunbury-on-Thames, Middlesex, TW16 6RG. For workshops and healing circles in Britain and countries outside Europe, contact New Life Promotions, 170 Campden Road, London, W8 7AS, tel: 0171 938 3788. For workshops and healing circles in Europe contact Walter Kraus, N-4532 Øslebø, Norway, tel: international code +47 382 87780.
• Transcendental Meditation: tel: 0171 402 3451
• THE NATURE CURE CLINIC, 15 Oldbury Place, London, W1M 3AL, tel: 0171 9352787.

The following resources are also mentioned in Part Three:

CHINESE MEDICAL CENTRE The Centres in Bath and Manchester provide information and consultations on acupuncture, massage, moxibustion, and traditional Chinese herbal therapy.

BATH: c/o Manvers Chambers, Manvers Street, Bath, BA1 1PE

tel: 01225 483393 fax: 01225 422037

MANCHESTER: c/o St John Chambers, 2 St John Street, Manchester, M3 4BD

tel: 0161 839 9283   fax: 0161 831 7956

See also Resources Part Four – acupuncture.

EDWARD BACH CENTRE For advice, information on Bach flower remedies, prepared treatment bottles, newsletter, and list of practitioners write to:

The Edward Bach Centre, Mount Vernon, Wallingford, Oxon, OX10 0PZ

FOOD & CHEMICAL ALLERGY ASSOCIATION

There is a booklet for £2 plus A5 s.a.e. available from:

27 Ferringham Lane, Ferring-by-sea, West Sussex, BN12 5NB.

Useful books for this section:

Brooke, Elizabeth, *A Woman's Book of Herbs*, The Women's Press, 1992, ISBN 0 7043 4296 0.

This book draws together astrology, herbal medicine, herbal lore, magic and spirituality. It has a useful glossary of terms, a list of herbal suppliers and a relevant reading list.

Curtis, Susan and Fraser, Romy, *Natural Healing For Women – Caring for Yourself with Herbs, Homeopathy & Essential Oils*, Pandora, 1991, ISBN 0 04 440645 2.

The authors are the founders of Neals Yard Remedies in London. The book has sections on the body's systems and their diseases; Materia Medica; and lifestyle. The appendices include a wide range of contacts and addresses for Britain, Australia and the USA; a cleansing diet; food charts on vitamins and minerals; and suggested reading.

Griggs, Barbara, *The Green Witch – A Modern Woman's*

Herbal, Vermillion, London, 1993, ISBN 0 7126 4725 2.
The book has sections on herbs around the home and kitchen, beauty care and remedies, including how to prepare herbal remedies, first aid and botanical names of herbs.
There is a full bibliography and a list of useful addresses of herbal and aromatherapy organisations and suppliers.

Harvey, Clare, and Cochrane, Amanda, *The Encyclopaedia of Flower Remedies – The Healing Power of Flower Essences from Around the World*, Thorsons, 1995, ISBN 0 7225 3096 X.
An international gathering together of information, including worldwide folk medicine. Extensive list of international addresses and courses, and a wide reading list.

McVicar, Jekka, *Jekka's Complete Herb Book*, Kyle Cathie Ltd, 1995, ISBN 1 85626 161 1.
Highly pictorial with a double page on each herb, history and medicinal and culinary uses. Includes growing instructions for pots, window boxes, back yards, small and large plots. Glossary of terms, reference section and short bibliography.

Weed, Susan, *The Menopausal Years the Wise Woman Way – Alternative Approaches for Women 30–90*, Ash Tree Publishing, Woodstock, New York, 1992, ISBN 9614620 4 3.
We have included this valuable book because of the confusion between menopause and ME. This is a source book for information on women's cycles and body rythms. Includes a useful glossary of terms, references and resources.

Part Four: Benefits, Rights and Beyond

BENEFITS

INCAPACITY ACTION – contact Kate Adams on 0181 533 2443. This pressure group was set up in response to changes in government legislation concerning invalidity benefit. The group has information on many aspects of benefits, including how to deal with the questionnaires for the All Work Test. Check with them and the Citizens' Advice

Bureau before going to your interview for the All Work Test or filling in any forms. Benefits information is also available from the ME Association and Action for ME.

If you also have to apply for housing benefit, you can ask advice from SHELTER. They are the experts on all aspects of housing advice and you do not have to be homeless for them to help you. The CAB and SHELTER addresses are in your local phone book.

DISABILITY AND RIGHTS

See Chapter 3 of *Lives Worth Living*, edited by Veronica Marris, Pandora, 1996, ISBN 0 04 440938 9.
Interviews with many women who have chronic illness including ME are combined here in this inspiring book.

Several contributors have recommended the following books and anthologies:

Disability Rights Handbook
Annually for Disability Alliance, tel: 0171 247 8776.
Gives current legislation advice and help with individual cases.

Keith, Lois (ed.), *Mustn't Grumble*, The Women's Press, 1994, ISBN 0 7043 4344 4.
Many of the issues that we deal with as women with ME are here voiced by many different women, whose lives have been changed by disability. Topics covered include family and friends, work and creativity, hope and despair, isolation and community.

Morris, Jenny, (ed.), *Able Lives*, The Women's Press, 1989, ISBN 0 7043 4155 7.
This book is about women's experience of paralysis following spinal cord injury. We include it here because it raises issues of other people's attitudes to disability which are very relevant to women's experiences of ME. It also discusses motherhood, wheelchairs, education and occupation, images, families and friends, growing older,

medical complications, pain, sexuality and relationships. It has an extensive resources and contacts list for women with disabilities, and a wide, general bibliography about women and disability.

From Anna's article on disability and ME the following books are also referred to:

Morris, Jenny, *Pride against Prejudice: A Personal Politics of Disability*, The Women's Press, 1991.

Morris, Jenny (ed.), *Encounters With Strangers: Feminism and Disability*, The Women's Press, 1996.

Swain, J, Finkelstein, V, French, S, and Oliver, M, (eds), *Disabling Barriers – Enabling Environments*, Sage Publications, 1993.

BEYOND CONVENTION

Homeopathy

a) The Society of Homeopaths, 2 Artizan Road, Northampton, NN1 4HU. Tel: 01604 214000. For an information leaflet and a register of practitioners, send a large s.a.e.
b) The UK Homeopathic Medical Association: for register send large s.a.e. to: UKHMA, 6 Livingstone Road, Gravesend, Kent, DA12, 5DZ. Tel: 01474 560336.

Contributors have suggested the following books on homeopathy:
Castro, Miranda, *The Complete Homeopathy Handbook*, Macmillan, 1990.
Vithoulkas, George, *The Science of Homeopathy* (this is comprehensive – check with your library for his other books as well).
Locke, Dr Andrew, *The Complete Guide to Homeopathy*, Dorling Kindersley.
Hayfield, Robin, *Homeopathy – A Practical Guide to Everyday Healthcare*, Gaia Books.

Acupuncture

Members of the British Acupuncture Council have completed a thorough training in traditional acupuncture, are bound by the Council's Codes of Ethics and Practice and are covered by Professional Indemnity and Public Liability insurance. A list of members in your area is available free of charge from The British Acupuncture Council, Park House, 206-208 Latimer Road, London, W10 6RE. Tel: 0181 964 0222.
See also resources on Traditional Chinese Medicine including Chinese herbs in Part Three.

Medical Herbalism

a) National Institute of Medical Herbalists
Send large s.a.e. to: 56 Longbrook Street, Exeter, Devon, EX4 6AH.
Tel: 01392 426022.
b) General Council and Register of Consultant Herbalists.
Send s.a.e. and four first-class stamps to:
32 King Edwards Road, Swansea, SA1 4LL.
Tel: 01792 655886.

For list of general books on herbs see Part Three.

International Resources

Addresses of ME organisations in other countries can be obtained from the ME Association and Action for ME.

Meg Torwl has compiled a resources list for New Zealand/Aotearoa. Anyone who would like a copy of this can contact the editor, with an international reply coupon, via the publisher.

Recommended Books published in New Zealand/Aotearoa:

Steincamp, Jaqueline, ME *Overload – Beating ME and CFIDS*, NZ, 1988.
This is an information and self-help book with chapters on symptoms and diet and several useful appendices.

Jeffreys, Toni, *The Mile High Staircase*, Hodder and Stoughton, 1982.
This autobiographical book by an ME sufferer is set in Australia.

Contributors' Notes

Kate Adams was born on 8 August 1954 and her early life was spent in Witchurch, Cardiff. She studied art at Kingston Polytechnic and completed the Postgraduate Art Teachers' Certificate in Brighton. She then went on to train as a social worker and, after qualifying, worked in Brighton and London. In 1988 she became ill with ME and was subsequently medically retired by her employers.

She currently lives in East London with her two cats. Since becoming ill she has started painting again and recently exhibited at Sutton House in Hackney and at Hackney Town Hall. She has also contributed to the magazines: *Disability Times*, *Disability Arts in London* and *Labour Left Briefing*. Due to cuts in resources and benefits paid to disabled people she has become involved in campaigning. In 1994, Incapacity Action was set up to fight for the repeal of the Incapacity for Work Act.

Ajay was born in London in 1953 to an Indian mother and English father. She went to school in Surrey and Sussex. She worked in the construction industry for nearly 15 years until going to university in 1989. She has lived in London since she was 15 and has known she was a lesbian since the age of 6. She has given up seeking a definition of herself that both suits her black friends and her white friends. She is of mixed racial heritage.

Aspen is white, technically in early middle age, but can feel anything from 0–696. She lives on the high edge of inter-connecting valleys west of the Pennines, surrounded and nourished by the beauty of the earth, but with no choice about having to interact with much ugliness created by human beings. She hopes many non-disabled people will find a cure for their chronically negative attitudes towards women with ME.

Kay Bastin is a white lesbian, feminist and activist/ hyperactivist. Born on 10 June 1954, she has been late ever since! After doing a Combined Arts degree at Leicester, she trained as a physiotherapist in Manchester, working for many years in the community until stopped in her tracks by ME in 1995. Still struggling with having to 'be' instead of 'do', she helps with *Eve's Back* (Manchester women's networking magazine) and writes poems and articles for *Eve's Back* and *Red Pepper* magazines amongst others.

Julia Cameron was born on 13 June 1952 in London. Her heritage is English/Scottish/Swiss. She studied psychology at Sheffield University and has a qualification in art therapy and training in counselling. However, her work life was almost entirely spent in community groups and the voluntary sector, mainly projects with a childcare/women's focus. Since getting ME she has been unable to work in structured employment, but was instrumental in setting up the North London ME Network, a self-help group for people with ME.

Kate Cargreaves was born in 1948 and raised in Sheffield. She has a psychology degree from Nottingham University, and has worked in various jobs in the statutory/voluntary caring sectors. She is the adoptive mother of two children and is a freelance writer. Her first book, *Journey To Our Children (Infertility and Adoption – One Couple's Moving Story)* was published in 1996. Among her other writings are a piece in The Women's Press anthology *A Stranger at My Table*, and articles in various publications including the *Guardian*, *Healing and Wholeness* and *New Generation*. Her short story *The Call* has just won a *Writer's Monthly* competition.

Parminder Chadha is an Indian of Punjabi origin from Kenya, East Africa. She came to England in 1963 at the age of three and a half and grew up in West London. She currently lives in Islington with her young son, Amer. She works intermittently now as a poetry and voice workshop tutor, and also as a researcher for the media and record industry. She hopes to return to performance this year and is keen to explore the experience of having ME in her work. She is active on the management committee of the North London ME network.

Rosie Chasseaud was born in 1946 in Liverpool and grew up in South London. She went to a convent school, then studied English and French at University. She has been a teacher, librarian, and much else. She has lived in Brighton since 1970, with time out in Aotearoa/New Zealand and the USA. Rosie has been studying studying embroidery and textiles, and loves music and gardening.

Kate Cook is a white, British radical feminist, born in Epsom, Surrey in 1960, but raised in Manchester and now firmly rooted there. She was a member of Manchester Rape Crisis and Manchester Women's Liberation Newsletter, and is now active within Manchester Justice for Women and Franki (Greater Manchester Women's Support Project). She is due to complete a degree in law in Summer 1997, health permitting.

Amanda Cornu was born in 1945 and is British and Canadian with French roots. She has lived in England for the last 20 years. She is a qualified social worker and worked for 25 years prior to being retired on health grounds, five years ago.

She also studied art and art history and has a degree in fine art. She has had poetry published in the magazines *First Time* and *The West in Her Eyes* and has also produced a booklet of her poems entitled *The Length of My Years*.

Fiona D'Alwis is from South-east Asia and spent her childhood in Brunei. She came to Britain to do her 'A' levels. After university she was mainly involved in community work.

She first became interested in alternative approaches to medicine when her daughter was born. She started looking at different approaches to health, and less well-known systems of medicine. She completed a four-year course in homeopathy, and is now registered with the Society of Homeopaths, having been in practice for the last six years. Fiona, her daughter, and her partner, live on the north coast of West Cornwall.

Linda Flynn was born on 7 September 1973 in Redbridge, Essex. She studied at Queen Mary and Westfield College, for a degree in English Literature and French. She has suffered from ME since November 1991.

She hopes to get involved in voluntary work for the Harold Wood Hospital in Essex, who provide an excellent unpaid service, which includes both diagnosis and advice for those with ME. She dedicates her article on ME to her family and friends who never doubted or questioned her illness, especially her mum, without whom her study at university would have been impossible.

Cordelia Galgut was born in Liverpool in 1955 and lived there until she was 12. She moved to London and has lived there mostly since then, currently in East London. She has been a teacher and worked in education for 16 years. For the last four years she has been training to be a counsellor and is now qualified.

Andrea Goodman was born in Hannover, Germany, in November 1962 to a German mother and Cornish father, who was an RAF policeman.

She has lived in Gloucestershire for the last 10 years. Before falling ill with ME she trained in a number of therapies and worked in this capacity. She now does some voluntary work on a telephone helpline and also a few hours of administrative work each week.

She is also studying Anthropology at Goldsmith's College in London. One of the biggest healing influences for her, besides the therapies, has been the support and encouragement of a few friends. She would like to thank Ros White, Jenny Daisley and Liz Willis for their joy in her successes.

Niki Green is a medical herbalist living and working in the far west of Cornwall. She was born in London in 1956 but grew up mostly in the country in Surrey. She studied social science and anthropology at Lancaster University in the 1970s and became interested in non-western medical traditions at that time. After successfully treating her own asthma and respiratory infections with herbs she decided to train as a medical herbalist. She has been a member of the National Institute of Medical Herbalists since 1988. Since then she has practised in London and in Cornwall – currently at the Natural Health Centre in Penzance.

Karon Hawes was born in Watford, Hertfordshire, in 1963, but has lived most of her life in Northamptonshire. She comes from a working-class background and identifies as a lesbian. She has had many jobs, ranging from catering, youth work, welfare rights and finally social work with adults with learning difficulties, until becoming ill with ME in March 1994.

Maria Jastrzębska was born in Warsaw, Poland, in 1953. She grew up in London and studied psychology at Sussex University. She has worked for a number of women's projects and has also been a teacher for many years. She is the author of *POSTCARDS FROM POLAND and other correspondences* (Working Press, 1991), with artist Jola Scicińska, and was one of the editors of *Forum Polek – The Polish Women's Forum*, a bilingual anthology. She has also contributed to various other anthologies, most recently *Musn't Grumble* (The Women's Press, 1994), and *As Girls Could Boast*, (Oscars Press, 1994). She lives in Brighton.

Evelyn McNally was born in Glasgow and is of strong, matriarchal Scots/Irish Catholic descent. She came to London at the age of 12. She trained as a playleader, and worked with the under-fives, mostly in the East End and Hackney. She studied for a Social Science degree at PCL (Political Science and Statistics), but considers that she has gained most of her education outside institutions. She has had poems published in *Magma 6* and *Magma 7*. She lives in London, a long stone's throw from Hampstead Heath.

Linda Newton was born in Leicester, the elder of twins, on 11 October 1952, with a condition diagnosed, at an early age, as spasticity. She was raised and still lives there, close to the city centre. She worked for the local authority for some 20 years and attained a middle-management post in housing.

In 1990, she trained to become a telephone 'helpline' volunteer at the local drug advisory centre. She would describe herself as a psychic/chocaholic/bisexual woman.

Lydia Nightingale lives on her own in her home town in Lancashire. In the past she has been a supermarket cashier, a librarian, a cleaner, a furniture restorer, an arts worker, a waitress and a painter and decorator. Nowadays she can be found doing the 'rituals' described in her article; getting actively involved in her local community centre; leading a limited social life; doing small-scale, home-based creative projects; and talking about joining a writing group.

Shelley Pielou was born in 1958 in Redhill, Surrey. She is a mixture of English, French and Irish and grew up in different countries in the Far East. She now lives in London. She went to drama school at 18 and worked as an actress in fringe and mainstream theatre, as well as doing bits of television work, films and commercials, until ME felled her in about 1991. She has now taken up painting and drawing, designs and sells greeting cards to raise money for charity and since contributing to this book has started participating in a creative writing class.

Lynda Poole was born in 1966 in Edgware, Middlesex. She grew up in Harrow, and now lives in Harlesden, north-west London. She has worked as a research assistant and as a clerical officer in the Civil Service. She would like to thank Bernadette Sheriff for being the model for Sandy's friend in her cartoons.

Anna Ravetz is British. Her mother is English, and her father originally an American Jew. She lived in Brighton and London for nine years, where she did a degree in history and became a legal advice worker. Her health broke down in 1988, when she became unable to work in a job. She did voluntary work from home, which included writing for and co-editing the journal *Action for ME*. She joined a group of disabled people working on access issues, developed an interest in gardening and garden design, and has done voluntary work in a local advice centre. She moved to Sheffield in 1990.

Elina Rigler was born in Finland in 1958 and also grew up there, but has lived in various parts of the UK for most of her adult life. She is currently living in north London. She did all types of casual work before embarking on a degree course in Linguistics at Essex University in 1982. At that time she enjoyed the academic life so much that she ended up working as a researcher, and subsequently obtained a PhD (also in Linguistics), at the University of Edinburgh.

Patricia Rock is a disabled, lesbian artist who has been living with a person with ME for 15 or 16 years, and has seen the hidden discrimination that people with ME experience. She is presently studying for a higher degree on women and disability.

Sue Sholl was born in Berkshire, the youngest of four children, in a working class family.
   She left school at 15 to do a year's college course in hotel reception and book-keeping, then moved to London, working

in the bill office of a big hotel.

Sue met her future husband when she was 18 and they were married when she was 21. She adopted his three small daughters as her own. After seven years, she fell pregnant, but in the early months of pregnancy, she contracted ME. It took seven years to get a diagnosis, by which time she had had her second baby. She is now learning to manage the illness better, and continues to enjoy an immensely rewarding family life.

Rebecca Shtasel was born in 1966 in Boston, Massachusetts. Her father's parents were Russian Jews, her mother's grandparents were German Lutherans and her parents emigrated with Rebecca to England when she was four year's old. She went to Leeds University to read English, and in 1990 she moved to Manchester where she gained a diploma in Youth and Community Work at Manchester Polytechnic. She then moved to London to become a youth worker and did advocacy and advice work for disability rights organisations, having an existing disability before developing ME. She is currently working on a book concerning ME. She lives in Brighton with her cat and four healthy flat-mates.

Marcia Francis Spence describes herself as a mother; godmother; companion; friend; survivor; pioneer; educator; writer; counsellor; mentor; traveller/explorer; graduate and life-long student.

Marcia's early years were spent in rural Jamaica. She then went to England and state education in Sheffield. She trained as a nurse before moving to Nottingham and subsequently to Durham, then full circle back to Sheffield. She is also an experienced probation officer, social worker, trainer and lecturer, and has written several academic papers. This paper is dedicated to her children, Ryan and Shane, and her circle of close friends.

Caroline Stedman was born in South London in a working class family in 1958. She grew up in that area and lives there again now. She has a degree in Social Psychology, and worked for seven years as a residential social worker with teenagers, gaining a social work training and MA along the way. Post ME she has begun training as a counsellor and now works part time for a national organisation which is concerned with teenagers and their sexual health. She is planning to train in psychotherapy as soon as funds allow so that she can have a wider scope to the way she works.

Sarah Thompson was born in an Essex village in 1967. She has lived in London since 1978. Straight from school she went to Botswana to teach English. She was about to study at the School of Oriental and African Studies when she contracted ME, aged 20. Despite being severely restricted she enjoys her garden, piano and poetry group.

Meg Torwl is a 30-year-old in-valid, middle-class pakeha of Scots/French ancestry. A twin, with multiple disabilities, she was born and lives in Aotearoa/New Zealand. She is a self-taught writer, photographer, and sometimes drawer, painter, collager, choreographer. She recently helped start a national newsletter for lesbians with disabilities.

Liz Tucker was born in 1963 in Worcestershire. She studied art and design at Hereford College, and then at Brighton for her degree. She later opted for a career as a businesswoman until 1993, when her life was devastated by illness. She is now recovering from ME and is determined to continue with writing, even if her only published work to date is a story about a witch and a Mars bar!

She now lives in Shropshire, with her husband and their miniature ponies, on the side of a hill where they have built their dream cottage.

Sharon Wachsler was born in Concord, Massachusetts in 1969. She is Jewish and a first-generation American. After receiving her BA in Sociology and Women's Studies from

Tufts University in 1992, Sharon became a self-defence instructor and an information and referral specialist for people with disabilities. In August of 1995 she became ill with CFIDS and MCS. Currently she spends her time resting, writing poetry, working for the rights of people with MCS, and cartooning. She lives in Somerville, MA with her two cats. Her essay 'Tied to the Railroad Tracks of Progress' will be published in the forthcoming Canadian Women's Press anthology *Bodies of Knowledge*.

Rita Wilcock was born in Norfolk in 1955 and grew up in Gloucestershire in a large working-class family. At the age of 18 she left home to go to art college in Manchester and now lives in Sheffield as a single parent of two daughters. She has identified as a lesbian since 1990.

Rita has had ME since summer 1993. She is now training with a voluntary counselling service for women which works with an awareness of women's differing cultures and oppressions. In summer 1996 she completed her degree course in Culture Studies after having had to defer course work for two years running due to ME.

Kate Wilson was born in Scotland in 1957. After university she went to London to study and became involved in the women's movement and gay politics. She also explored therapy and alternative medicine, eventually training in Traditional Chinese Medicine and psycho-dynamic counselling. After living and practising for 13 years in Hackney, she decided to move to Cornwall, near Land's End. She runs a women's B&B and organises creative healing residential workshops. She also continues to practise acupuncture and to make sculpture.

Abigail Wright was born in 1978 in South Yorkshire and still lives there with her family. She worked at a Fine Art Auction House and was accepted for university to gain qualifications to become an antique valuer and auctioneer.

Valerie Wright was born in South Yorkshire in 1949 to British parents. She spent her early years in the West Riding, where she still lives. She is a Registered General Nurse and has studied part time as a mature student for an Advanced Diploma in Counselling. She has been nursing in family planning and women's health for many years. She has two daughters in higher education.